TOTAL HEART HEALTH

How to Prevent and Reverse Heart Disease
with the Maharishi Vedic Approach to Health

ROBERT H. SCHNEIDER, M.D., F.A.C.C.,
AND JEREMY Z. FIELDS, PH.D.

T0273790

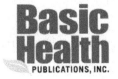

Basic
Health
PUBLICATIONS, INC.

The information contained in this book is based upon the research and personal and professional experiences of the authors. It is not intended as a substitute for consulting with your physician or other healthcare provider. Any attempt to diagnose and treat an illness should be done under the direction of a healthcare professional.

The publisher does not advocate the use of any particular healthcare protocol but believes the information in this book should be available to the public. The publisher and authors are not responsible for any adverse effects or consequences resulting from the use of the suggestions, preparations, or procedures discussed in this book. Should the reader have any questions concerning the appropriateness of any procedures or preparation mentioned, the authors and the publisher strongly suggest consulting a professional healthcare advisor.

®Transcendental Meditation, TM-Sidhi, Maharishi Vedic Approach to Health, Maharishi Consciousness-Based Health Care, Maharishi Ayurveda, Maharishi Rejuvenation Program, Maharishi Amrit Kalash, Maharishi Vedic Organic Agriculture, Maharishi Vedic, Maharishi Sthapatya Veda, Maharishi Yoga, Maharishi Yagya, Maharishi Vedic Astrology, Maharishi Jyotish, Maharishi Gandharva Veda, Maharishi Gandharva Veda music, Maharishi Vedic Sound, Maharishi Vedic Vibration Technology, Consciousness-Based, Maharishi University of Management, Maharishi School of the Age of Enlightenment, Maharishi Vedic Health Center, Maharishi Peace Palace, Maharishi Enlightenment Center are registered or common law trademarks licensed to Maharishi Vedic Education Development Corporation and used under sublicense or with permission.

Basic Health Publications, Inc.
28812 Top of the World Drive • Laguna Beach, CA 92651 • 949-715-7327

Library of Congress Cataloging-in-Publication Data
Schneider, Robert H.
    Total heart health : how to prevent and reverse heart disease with the maharishi vedic approach to health / by Robert H. Schneider and Jeremy Z. Fields.—1st ed.
        p. cm.
    Includes bibliographical references and index.
        ISBN-13: 978-1-59120-087-1
        ISBN-10: 1-59120-087-3
    1. Heart—Diseases—Prevention. 2. Medicine, Ayurvedic. I. Fields, Jeremy Z. II. Title.
        RC682.S275   2006
        616.1'205—dc22

                                                        2006003930

Editor: Cheryl Hirsch • Copyeditor: Carol Rosenberg
Typesetting/Book design: Gary A. Rosenberg • Cover design: Mike Stromberg

Printed in the United States of America

10   9   8   7   6   5   4   3   2   1

To Maharishi Mahesh Yogi

Whose unbounded compassion and energy
for the benefit of humanity and total
knowledge of health and natural law
are inspiring the people of all nations
to reconstruct the whole world to create a
disease-free society and heaven on earth.

The problem of health is the most vital problem of life. Everything depends upon health. The peace and happiness of man within himself, his accomplishments in different spheres of life, his attitude and behavior with others, and above all, the very significance of his existence depend upon health.

In order to consider health fully we should take into account the health of the individual and that of the cosmos—man and his atmosphere.

—MAHARISHI MAHESH YOGI
IN *THE SCIENCE OF BEING AND ART OF LIVING,* 1963

To Maharishi Mahesh Yogi

*Whose unbounded compassion and energy
for the benefit of humanity and total
knowledge of health and natural law
are inspiring the people of all nations
to reconstruct the whole world to create a
disease-free society and heaven on earth.*

*The problem of health is the most vital problem of life.
Everything depends upon health. The peace and happiness of
man within himself, his accomplishments in different spheres
of life, his attitude and behavior with others, and above all,
the very significance of his existence depend upon health.*

*In order to consider health fully we should take into
account the health of the individual and that of
the cosmos—man and his atmosphere.*

—MAHARISHI MAHESH YOGI
IN *THE SCIENCE OF BEING AND ART OF LIVING,* 1963

Contents

Acknowledgments

Making the Total Heart Health program available to the public has been the fulfillment of a long-time desire, and we have many people to thank for helping us conceive, develop, and write this book.

First and foremost, we would like to express our sincere and deep gratitude to Maharishi Mahesh Yogi, who revived this knowledge from the ancient Vedic civilization of India and brought it to the modern world in a scientific framework.

We express special gratitude to Professor Tony Nader, M.D., Ph.D., now honored with the title Maharaja Nader Raam, for his noble discovery of the Veda and Vedic literature in the human physiology and for his leadership of the Global Country of World Peace. Professor Nader is the ideal physician-scientist-teacher-leader.

We express heartfelt appreciation to our fellow scientists, physicians, and teachers who have paved the way before us and have acted graciously as role models and mentors for us for thirty-five years. These pioneers of the new age of medicine and health care include Dr. Robert Keith Wallace, Founding President of Maharishi University of Management; the late Dr. Charles Alexander, our original partner in research at the Institute for Natural Medicine and Prevention; Dr. David Orme-Johnson; Dr. Barry Charles; Dr. Stuart Rothenberg; Dr. Richard Averbach; Dr. Hari Sharma; Dr. Nancy Lonsdorf; and Dr. Manohar Palakurti—all of whom have been role models, teachers, colleagues, and friends. We are grateful to Dr. Bevan Morris, President of Maharishi University of Management, for his ongoing support, inspiration, and leadership. Dr. Craig Pearson, Executive Vice President of the University, provided continual encouragement.

We also wish to acknowledge the groundbreaking contributions and leadership of Dr. John Hagelin, Director of the Institute of Science, Technology and

Public Policy, for his pioneering research on the unified field of natural law and its applications to consciousness, health, and peace.

Maharishi Ayurveda Products International and its Council of Maharishi Ayurveda Physicians generously provided much resource material on the physiological approaches of the Total Heart Health program.

We are indebted to Mary Zeilbeck and Sherry Hogue for their editing, research, and organizing expertise and outstanding contributions. Dr. Steven Schneider collaborated with us on the conception of this book many years ago. This finished work would not have been created without their capable skills, knowledge, and enthusiasm. We are grateful to our patient and energetic agent, Joelle Delbourgo, to our committed publisher, Norman Goldfind, and to our untiring and talented editor, Cheryl Hirsch.

We wish to acknowledge the foresight, vision, and generous financial support of the Retirement Research Foundation, its Board of Trustees and officers, particularly Marilyn Hennessy and Dr. Brian Hofland, Jeffrey Abramson and the Abramson Family Foundation, and the National Institutes of Health (NIH), National Heart, Lung and Blood Institute, and National Institute on Aging. The preparation of this book was supported in part by a Specialized Center of Research (SCOR) grant number P50AT00082 from the NIH-National Center for Complementary and Alternative Medicine. Its contents are solely the responsibility of the authors and do not necessarily represent the official views of the NIH or private foundations.

We are grateful to our scientific colleagues and administrative team at the Institute for Natural Medicine and Prevention at Maharishi University of Management for their unerring service, energy, knowledge, and organization that formed the basis for much of this book. These exceptional individuals include Dr. Sanford Nidich, Dr. Carolyn King, Dr. John Salerno, Dr. Maxwell Rainforth, Dr. Kenneth Walton, Linda Heaton, Jean Symington Craig, Laura Alcorn, and others who worked with us over the years. And, to dear friend, Celia Bella.

Lastly, we honor the memory of our parents, who supported and encouraged us throughout our lives and supplied the foundation for becoming the best we could be to contribute to a healthier and more peaceful world.

Awakening the Body's Inner Intelligence

I f you are one of the 150 million Americans who suffer from heart disease or one of its major risk factors, such as high blood pressure, high cholesterol, obesity, stress, or diabetes, this book is for you. If you are concerned about developing heart disease because a close member of your family had a heart attack or stroke (as nearly one in every two Americans will), this book is also for you. Whether you want to prevent this debilitating and possibly deadly condition or reverse it in yourself or in a family member or loved one, this book will offer you a completely new understanding and practical approach that will create a major transformation in your health and total well-being.

HEART DISEASE: AN UNCHECKED EPIDEMIC

Today, heart disease has reached epidemic proportions. It is now the leading cause of death in the United States and throughout the world. It is estimated that nearly half the people in this country will die prematurely because of this disease. Already, 65 million Americans suffer from high blood pressure, a common precursor to heart disease. Unfortunately, conventional medicine has been largely unable to prevent this epidemic despite the tens of billions of dollars spent over the last fifty years on research to develop better diagnostic tests and treatments. Moreover, the hazardous side effects of modern drugs and surgical procedures used to treat heart disease and other diseases now rank as the third-leading cause of death in America. Clearly, modern medicine has not lived up to its promise to eliminate heart disease and, in the eyes of many, is failing.

But why? Because modern medicine has failed to locate the ultimate cause of heart disease and does not operate at this most fundamental level of human health. Because modern heart medicine works on relatively superficial levels. Because modern cardiology focuses on fixing or replacing the "parts" of a person, such as diseased arteries, instead of on reversing the imbalances at the root of the disease, imbalances that affect all the arteries in the body. The conventional approach to heart disease treats you as a collection of tubes and valves—albeit a highly sophisticated collection with switches and feedback mechanisms—but ignores you as a whole person. It also ignores your individual mind-body type.

With a limited approach, one gets limited results. That is, it may be possible to suppress your symptoms of chest pain or to lower your high blood pressure or high cholesterol levels with drugs, but if you stop taking the drugs, the symptoms of high blood pressure or high cholesterol or heart disease come right back. Furthermore, you may have endured many unpleasant and often harmful side effects of these drugs or surgery unnecessarily, when you could have been reversing—or better yet preventing—the disease at its source, and doing so naturally.

Based on twenty-five years of clinical research into the basic causes of cardiovascular diseases and the most effective means to prevent and treat them (Robert Schneider, M.D., F.A.C.C.) and more than thirty years of research in neuroscience and human physiology (Jeremy Fields, Ph.D.), we can safely say that, if you are interested in achieving total heart health, the conventional medical approach to prevention and treatment of heart disease will not adequately work for you.

A WAY OUT OF THE DILEMMA

As someone who is seeking ways to combat or prevent heart disease effectively and without harmful side effects, you should not give up hope in the face of these staggering statistics and clinical facts about heart disease because a powerful source of intelligence and healing is available to you. Indeed, this level is deep within you, underlying your mind and body. And it is easy to gain access to it and benefit from it.

As discussed more thoroughly in Chapter 4, this source is your body's own *inner intelligence.* The principles and practices of the Maharishi Vedic Approach to Health℠ allow you to gain access to this source of intelligence and reestablish the flow of biological intelligence within your body. As balance is increasingly reestablished in your physiology with these approaches, the results will be both healing and preventive.

The ancient Vedic scientists, also called *rishis* or seers, viewed this inner intelligence as a field of unbounded energy and intelligence, a unified field of natural law that gives rise to everything else in the universe. At first this may sound unfamiliar to you. However, this concept, which was cognized ages ago in the Vedic civilization of ancient India, has been lively in modern science, especially modern physics, for many decades. It may surprise you to learn that modern physics, has, over the last 100 years or so, developed a view of the unified field that completely corroborates the ancient Vedic view. Modern science has come to understand that the unified field is the source of all of the particles and forces of nature and therefore is literally at the basis of everything in the universe.

Discovery of the Unified Field by Modern Science

Over the past 300 years, modern science has progressively uncovered deeper layers of order in nature. Quantum physicists, scientists involved in the branch of physics that studies and predicts the properties of physical systems at subatomic levels and even smaller, have determined that all the known forces in nature can be described in terms of just four main forces called *quantum fields.* These four fundamental forces are the electromagnetic field, the weak field, the strong field, and the gravitational field.

The electromagnetic field generates heat, light, radio waves, and many other frequencies of electromagnetic radiation. The weak and strong forces hold atoms together, and the gravitational field is gravity, which anchors objects to the ground. These four forces combine and interact with one another to form a cohesive structure for all the forces and elementary particles that make up physical systems, including our bodies, plants, rocks, planets, solar systems, galaxies, and the whole universe. Gradually, quantum physicists have come to understand that these fundamental fields are simply different aspects, or vibrational modes, of a single unified field of natural law. (See Figure 1 on page 4.)

Since the unified field is at the basis of all the fundamental forces and particles of the natural world, it is also at the basis of the laws of physics, chemistry, biology, and human physiology. This is why the ancients called this level *the inner intelligence of the body.* This brings us to the main point of the Maharishi Vedic Approach to Health: its diagnostic and therapeutic approaches function on the level of the unified field, which is the deepest level of your own physiology. Thus, while this book is not primarily about physics, it is about total heart health, yet the two are intimately related. In order to understand the basis of both heart disease and heart health, you need to understand the basis of human physiology. Later on, we will describe how the Maharishi Vedic Approach to Health is unified field-based health care and how this knowledge can be used to prevent heart disease and restore complete health in ways that conventional medicine cannot.

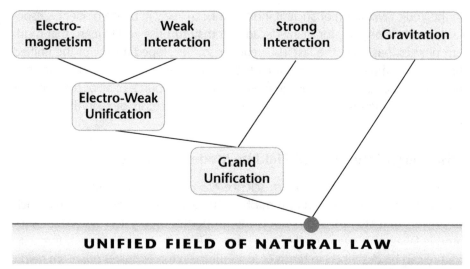

Figure 1. The Relationship of the Four Fundamental Forces of Nature to the Unified
         Field of All the Laws of Nature

THE ORIGINS OF THE MAHARISHI VEDIC
APPROACH TO HEALTH

Vedic science is an age-old tradition of knowledge that has its origins in the
ancient Vedic civilization of India. Many thousands of years ago, the scientists
of the Vedic tradition discovered, through explorations of their own highly
developed inner awareness, a unified field from which all the laws of nature
emerge. They discovered that this field is at the basis of human consciousness,
mind, and body. In the Vedic language of Sanskrit, the unified field is called
Atma, which means the "the innermost self of everyone."

This knowledge and the practical applications or technologies of the unified field have been passed down from teacher to student for as long as records
of human knowledge exist, and are now considered to be the oldest continuous tradition of knowledge in the world. Although it is primarily an oral tradition, this knowledge was written down in a large collection of verses and books
known as the Veda. In Sanskrit, *Veda* means "knowledge." The Veda is divided
into forty disciplines or branches, collectively referred to as the Vedic literature.
Each branch specializes in a particular aspect of the traditional knowledge of the
unified field of natural law and its practical applications.

While being passed down from generation to generation over the centuries,
this original knowledge eventually became fragmented and many of its key elements became lost. The traditional Vedic approach to health came to be practiced without knowledge of its source—the unified field of natural law and the

inner intelligence inherent in the person. Fortunately, over the last fifty years, working together with the foremost Vedic physicians and experts of India, Maharishi Mahesh Yogi—who is considered the leading Vedic scholar and teacher in the world today and is the founder of the Transcendental Meditation® program—restored the missing knowledge. He revived and systematized this knowledge in a scientific, practical, and easy-to-use framework. He formulated a science and technology of the unified field that restores the ancient unified field-based approach to total health.

Using the Maharishi Vedic Approach to Health to Prevent and Reverse Heart Disease

The Maharishi Vedic Approach to Health is a sophisticated system of prevention-oriented natural health care derived from the ancient and authentic texts of the Veda. The contemporary application of this knowledge to prevent and reverse heart disease and restore complete heart health is the Total Heart Health program. Our fifty years of combined professional experience involving scientific research, clinical practice, and teaching the Maharishi Vedic Approach to Health, as well as the experiences of millions of people worldwide who have used these modalities, form the basis of this program. Each of the forty approaches of the Maharishi Vedic Approach to Health is based on one of the forty major divisions of the Vedic literature. Each of these approaches includes practical techniques to restore the connection of your mind and body to your inner intelligence, the unified field of all the laws of nature within you.

For simplicity in this book, the forty branches of the ancient Vedic approach to health are integrated and divided into the three major domains of influence on your health: mind, body, and environment. Balance in all of these areas is required for total heart health. The methods of the Maharishi Vedic Approach to Health restore balance through diagnostic and therapeutic approaches that work through these three spheres of influences. Despite the differences among the approaches within these three major domains, they have in common the ability to enliven the connection of an individual to his or her inner intelligence. Total heart health is possible only when the influences that affect your mind, body, and environment are considered together, and all in terms of connecting back to your body's inner healer.

The practical benefits of this new approach to heart disease have been verified by more than 600 published scientific studies conducted at 200 independent universities and research institutes in thirty countries around the world. In particular, research studies performed at our research institute, the Institute for Natural Medicine and Prevention at Maharishi University of Management in collaboration with several major academic medical centers, have shown that the

Total Heart Health program results in significant health benefits. These include substantial and long-lasting reductions in high blood pressure, reduced need for blood pressure medications, and reductions in high cholesterol, smoking, psychological stress, and drug abuse. Further, studies published in major medical journals indicate slowing or reversal of hardening of the arteries, and an increase in life span in long-term participants in the Total Heart Health program. The results of this scientific research on the Total Heart Health program have been reported widely in the popular media in several thousand television, radio, magazine, and newspaper stories that have made their way around the world. Now for the first time, this program is available to the general public in this book, *Total Heart Health.*

HOW TO USE THIS BOOK

This book is designed to give you the most up-to-date knowledge and practical guidelines for achieving total heart health. It should serve as a manual to help you fill in the gaps not provided by conventional medicine and may help to prevent or reduce your need for drugs or surgery. However, the information contained here is not intended to replace the care of your medical doctor. Rather, it provides you with options to consider that may be used to complement conventional care. If you already have heart disease, high blood pressure, or one or more of the other major risk factors for heart disease, we recommend that you discuss this program with your doctor before you make any changes.

You may choose to try one, several, or all of the approaches in the Total Heart Health program. The choice is yours. Research indicates that each approach provides distinct health benefits, but that using several or all of the approaches together creates a synergy that multiplies the program's beneficial effects. As you read on, here's what you can expect to learn:

Section I describes the widespread epidemic of heart disease. It presents the conventional view of the causes of heart disease and its major risk factors and their traditional treatments. This section of the book demonstrates the pressing need for a new and effective program for heart disease—a bold new angle to heart disease, one that not only addresses the problem, but also can prevent it and provide you with the means to achieve good health. Section II is devoted to the Total Heart Health program. We open this section with a description of the knowledge and technologies of the Maharishi Vedic Approach to Health on which the Total Heart Health program is based; then, we briefly introduce the program itself. As noted previously, the Total Heart Health program utilizes the three major domains of influence on your health according to the Maharishi Vedic Approach to Health—mind, body, and environment—to provide natural, scientifically proven, side-effect-free solutions to heart disease and its major risk factors. The remainder of the book is divided into three parts with each part devoted to an approach based on one of the three domains.

Part One focuses on the Mind Approach. The Transcendental Meditation® program is a cornerstone of the Maharishi Vedic Approach to Health. This is a simple, natural, technique for gaining profound rest in mind and body and enlivening the body's inner intelligence. The remarkable effects this program has on reducing stress and improving health, especially heart disease and its risk factors, are presented here along with a description of the practice of the Transcendental Meditation technique.

Part Two presents the Body Approach. It gives an overview of physiology and the causes of heart disease from the perspective of the Maharishi Vedic Approach to Health. It provides you with practical, easy-to-use recommendations for preventing heart disease and its risk factors through diet, exercise, and your daily routine.

In Part Three, we describe the Environment Approach of the program and explain the effects of the environment, both near and far. The near environment includes your home and physical surroundings, as well as the collective consciousness of the society in which you live. The far environment includes the planets and stars and the effects they can have on your heart and overall health. Later in Part Three, we provide guidelines for taking advantage of the natural rhythms and cycles in nature and using the Vedic sound programs for preventing heart disease and promoting health.

The Epilogue offers a final word on using the multiple approaches of the Maharishi Vedic Approach to Health in an integrated way to create total heart health and a vision for the future of health for everyone.

I. The Conventional Causes and Treatments of Heart Disease and Its Risk Factors

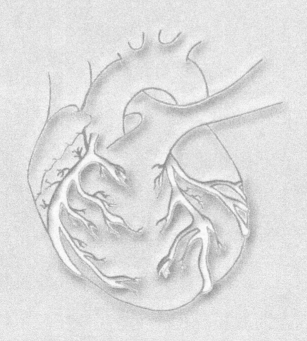

♥ CHAPTER 1 ♥

The Epidemic of Modern Society

HEART DISEASE IS THE NUMBER-ONE THREAT to your health today. Having reached epidemic proportions, heart disease now accounts for more deaths in the United States and other developed countries than the next sixteen causes of death combined. The American Heart Association estimates that 1.1 million Americans will experience a heart attack this year. Of these, more than 500,000 will die suddenly, without warning. Even those who manage to survive usually won't escape the ravages of the disease, which can cripple and dramatically diminish their quality of life and the lives of those who love and depend on them. Moreover, the many risk factors that lurk under the surface, slowly advancing this disease, are like stealth bombers, often not giving us a warning until it is too late.

This chapter describes the extent and gravity of the epidemic and describes the healthy cardiovascular system and the step-by-step progression of events leading to atherosclerosis (accumulation in blood vessels of fatty plaques) and, ultimately, to the diagnosis of full-fledged heart disease. Understanding the heart and vascular system and what can go wrong with this exquisitely synchronized network is a prerequisite for understanding the deeper causes of heart disease from the perspective of the Maharishi Vedic Approach to Health, and the treatment and preventive approaches for total heart health that are discussed in Section II.

To better understand both the modern and Vedic approaches to heart disease, it is useful to have some understanding about the anatomy and physiology of both the normal and the diseased cardiovascular system. We start by briefly describing the healthy cardiovascular system and then discuss what happens when it is not so healthy.

THE HEALTHY CARDIOVASCULAR SYSTEM

Your cardiovascular system has the indispensable role of feeding every one of the approximately 600 billion cells in your body. It is a system that consists of a pump and a network of elastic tubes through which fluid circulates throughout the body. The pump, of course, is the heart, which works 24/7, never pausing for more than a second. The elastic tubes are the circulatory system, a network made up of 60,000 miles of blood vessels, ranging in size from the arteries, which are large enough to carry six to seven quarts of blood every minute, to the capillaries, which allow only one tiny blood cell through at a time. The fluid is the circulating blood, which transports oxygen and vital nutrients to every cell in the body, including heart cells. As blood circulates, it also picks up waste products from the body tissues, which are then eliminated with the help of the kidneys, liver, and lungs. The flow of blood throughout the body's 60,000 miles of blood vessels takes fewer than ninety seconds. Without the constant functioning of your cardiovascular system, your cells would no longer have the nutrients or the supply of oxygen needed to keep your body functioning, and you would die in less than a minute.

The Healthy Heart

Your heart is a pump made of muscle. Although it is only a little bigger than your fist, it generates the driving force that delivers nutrients and oxygen through the blood to every cell in the body. Every day, the heart beats (expands and contracts) approximately 100,000 times as it pumps nearly 2,000 gallons of blood through your circulatory system. The two sides of the heart are completely dedicated to this purpose. The right side receives oxygen-depleted blood from the body and transports it to the lungs where it picks up oxygen that you have breathed in. This oxygen-rich blood leaves the lungs and returns to the left side of the heart where it is then pumped outward into the rest of the body.

Each side of the heart muscle consists of two chambers: an upper chamber, or atrium, which receives the blood from the body through the veins, and a lower chamber, the ventricle, which pumps blood out into the body through the arteries. The result is a sequence of perfectly organized contractions of the four chambers. The sequence starts when the right atrium of the heart collects the bluish oxygen-depleted blood from the body, and then squeezes it down into the right ventricle. When the ventricle is full, it contracts to force the blood out to the lungs, where the blood is oxygenated. The upper left atrium collects the bright red, newly oxygenated blood and squeezes it down into the left ventricle, which then contracts and pumps the blood out into the entire body. Because the left ventricle of the heart is responsible for delivering blood throughout the body, it is stronger and larger than the right ventricle, which only pumps blood to the lungs.

The Heart's Assistants

This entire process is assisted by an electrical system, which precisely orchestrates the sequence of contractions of the different chambers of the heart. The heart's natural pacemaker, called the *sino-atrial node,* triggers each set of contractions, which are coordinated to the millisecond by special fibers of the electrical system of the heart.

Also helping the functioning of the four chambers of the heart muscle is a set of four valves: tricuspid, pulmonary, mitral, and aortic valves. Much like the lock gates of the Panama Canal that open and close in sequence to direct the flow of water and ships between the Atlantic and Pacific Oceans, these valves open and close in perfect sequence to direct the flow of blood from the veins of the body through the chambers of the heart and then back out into the arteries of the body. Of the four valves that direct the flow of blood, the tricuspid and mitral valves have the inside job of controlling the flow of blood between the atria and the ventricles of the heart. The pulmonary and aortic valves control the flow of blood between the heart and the rest of the body.

The Healthy Circulatory Network

The channels of elastic tubes that connect the heart with the lungs and the rest of the body are of paramount importance to the heart's role of distributing nutrients and oxygen to the body, including to the heart itself. These tubes are called *arteries, veins,* and *capillaries,* and they make up your circulatory system. They are the second major part of the cardiovascular system (the heart is the first), forming an enormous network throughout your body.

The arteries are the channels that take blood from the heart and distribute it to the body. They are large vessels with thick, elastic walls. The two main arteries of the body are the aorta and the pulmonary artery. The pulmonary artery carries oxygen-depleted blood from the heart to the lungs. After the lungs oxygenate the blood and send it back to the heart, the aorta, which is the largest artery of the body, guides the oxygen-rich blood from the heart out to the rest of the body. The aorta is able to supply blood to the body with the help of other arteries, which branch out until they become small arterioles. These smaller vessels bring the blood to a vast network of capillaries, which eventually end up being microscopic and not much wider than the size of a single cell. It is at this point that the system is fine enough to feed the individual cells that make up the tissues of the body.

Veins bring blood back from the body to the heart. The largest veins in the body are called the *venae cavae.* These include the superior vena cava, which receives blood from the head and arms, and the inferior vena cava, which receives blood from the abdomen and legs. Blood from the superior and inferior venae cavae is collected in the heart, where it is then driven out into the lungs for oxygenation. The pulmonary vein then takes the blood from the lungs back to the heart, which then sends it out on its next journey through the rest of the body.

The network of veins is the mirror image of the network of arteries. Veins like arteries branch out into increasingly smaller vessels father away from the heart. The blood in the veins flows from the small vessels in the periphery into increasingly larger vessels in the center of the body. The blood eventually empties into the largest veins, the venae cavae, and then returns back to the heart for recirculation in the arteries. The structure of the heart and its major blood vessels is illustrated in Figure 1.1.

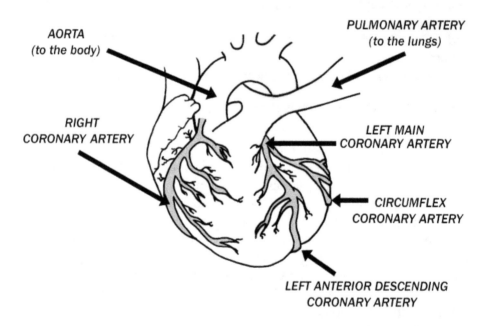

Figure 1.1. The Heart and the Coronary Arteries

The Coronary Arteries

Your heart cannot directly use the nutrients and oxygen from the blood that passes through its four chambers. In order to obtain the nutrients and oxygen the heart needs from the blood, it relies on the coronary arteries, the first arteries to branch off from the aorta. There are two coronary arteries: the right coronary artery and the left main coronary artery. These arteries branch out and wrap around the exterior of the heart muscle.

The left main coronary artery, which is on the left side of the heart, divides into two branches: the left anterior descending coronary artery, which supplies blood to the front of the heart, and the left circumflex coronary artery, which wraps around the left side of the heart to the back where it supplies blood to the left part of the heart. The right coronary artery, on the right side of the heart, feeds the right part of the heart. From these arteries, smaller blood vessels diverge into the deeper layers of the heart muscle.

Because the coronary arteries are the sole pathways used to feed the heart, they are critical to the health of the heart muscle. Indeed, a blockage in one of these arteries is the most common cause of heart disease. Heart attacks, angina pectoris, heart failure, or sudden cardiac death (cardiac arrest) all originate from blockages in these vessels due to atherosclerosis (accumulation of fatty plaques), or formation of a blood clot (thrombosis). A blockage in the left main coronary artery is especially troubling because it is a major artery feeding several arterial branches that serve the heart, particularly the left ventricle, which is responsible for pumping blood throughout the body. Figure 1.2 below illustrates the difference between a healthy artery and a clogged artery.

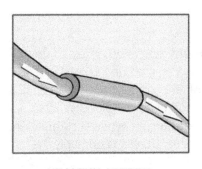 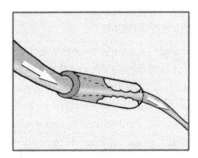

HEALTHY ARTERY   **BLOCKED ARTERY**

Figure 1.2. Comparison of a Healthy Artery and a Diseased Coronary Artery

WHAT IS HEART DISEASE?

Many different ideas probably come to mind when you try to define the term *heart disease.* We frequently hear the terms *heart attack* (an interruption of blood flow to the heart muscle) and *heart failure* (an inability of the heart muscle to pump an adequate amount of blood), and may think of these first. Or you may think about a loved one or someone you know who just had a heart valve replacement, an operation in which a diseased valve is replaced by an artificial one. Perhaps you have experienced fluttering or palpitations in your heart and worried you might be experiencing an arrhythmia (irregular rhythm of the heart) due to damage to the heart's pacemaker. Then there is hypertension, also called *high blood pressure,* a common precursor not only to coronary heart disease, but also to hypertensive heart disease, a disorder involving the enlargement of the heart muscle caused by prolonged and uncontrolled high blood pressure. There is also congenital heart disease, a heart malformation present at birth, and a host of other conditions that are rare but still problematic.

Although technically the term *heart disease* encompasses a wide range of conditions, for the purposes of this book, only its most common form has been chosen for our focus: *coronary heart disease* caused by atherosclerosis of the coronary arteries. The reason for this choice is simple. Coronary heart disease is the leading form of heart disease in the world. It is the most serious—taking more lives than any other health problem—and is at the root of many of the other major heart diseases we just mentioned. Coronary heart disease is the blocking of the coronary arteries, the heart's lifeline to the nutrients and oxygen it needs to work. And this blockage is due to atherosclerosis, a chronic and debilitating process that clogs, narrows, hardens, and damages the nutrient- and oxygen-supplying arteries of the heart responsible for keeping it, and you, alive.

Atherosclerosis

So, what exactly is atherosclerosis? The term *atherosclerosis* refers to the thickening and hardening of the artery walls caused by the buildup of plaque in the inner lining of the arteries. Plaque is a combination of fatty substances, cholesterol, fibrous tissue, decaying muscle cells, blood platelets (blood-cell fragments important in clotting), calcium, and other substances. While accumulation of plaque can occur anywhere in the vascular system, it affects primarily the large- and medium-sized arteries that feed the brain and the heart. This includes the two major arteries on either side of the neck that carry blood to the brain known as the *carotid arteries.* It also includes: 1) the elastic arteries, like the aorta, which accepts blood pumped out of the heart through the aortic valve and transports the blood, and the large quantities of vital nutrients and oxygen it contains, to the entire body, and 2) the muscular arteries, like the coronary arteries, which feed these essential substances to the heart cells to keep them functioning properly.

With the buildup of plaque and the onset of atherosclerosis in the blood vessels of the body, everything changes. Without your noticing, processes leading toward degeneration of your heart and other vital organs take place. It doesn't happen overnight, but rather progresses silently, gradually developing over the years, slowly taking its toll. Arteries that were once supple and strong become increasingly narrow and hard, incrementally restricting the flow of oxygen and nutrients to the body, until one day, the flow in one or more coronary arteries is seriously blocked, or even stops completely.

Just as you need to have oxygen and nutrients to live, the cells of the heart need oxygen and vital nutrients to live. When complete blockage of blood flow in an artery occurs, the tissues fed by that artery become deprived of oxygen and nutrients. As a result, the area of the heart or brain, kidneys, extremities, or other organ that was fed by that artery dies. If a sufficient area of the organ dies, then the organ dies. If that organ is the heart, then you die too.

When the blockage takes place in the heart, it's called a *heart attack;* when the blood supply to the brain is blocked, it is called a *stroke.* Because of these serious and potentially deadly consequences, particularly to the body's critical organs and systems, atherosclerosis must be treated, and more important, prevented. Atherosclerosis is responsible for the top two causes of death worldwide: heart attack, also called *myocardial infarction* (MI); and stroke, also called *cerebrovascular accident* (CVA), which results in the sudden death of all or part of the brain.

To understand more fully how atherosclerosis develops, it is useful to know more about the arteries. Arteries are carefully constructed for carrying out their essential role in the body. To do this, the artery has three layers. The outer layer is a strong protective covering composed of connective tissue, collagen, and elastic fibers called the *adventitia.* It holds the artery together, yet allows it to constrict and expand as needed, and connects it to the rest of your body. Just inside the adventitia is a central, thicker layer known as the *media.* This layer consists of muscle cells and elastic fibers, which give the artery the elasticity to control the diameter of the opening of the blood vessel, and thereby regulate how much blood circulates through the vessel. The third and innermost layer of the artery is the *intima.* The lining of the intima's elastic membrane is covered by a single layer of cells called the *endothelium.* The endothelium gives the artery its flat smooth inner surface along which the blood can flow easily, and like a general, it directs many of the actions the artery takes to protect itself and fulfill its purpose in getting oxygen and nutrients to your body. The hollow center of the artery through which the blood flows is called the *lumen.*

It is in the inner layer of the artery, the *intima,* where the main drama of atherosclerosis takes place. Other parts of the artery may participate in secondary ways, such as remodeling themselves and sending protective cells to the inner intima layer in order to keep the center of the artery open for the passage of blood to the body.

How Atherosclerosis Develops

Although modern medicine's understanding of how atherosclerosis develops is limited, the disease is thought to be triggered by a combination of factors. Some are external factors such as dietary cholesterol, stress, and cigarette smoke; others are internal factors such as the abnormal activation of your artery's own internal repair and protective mechanisms, which can cause excess inflammation. Damage due to internal factors tends to occur at areas of strain, such as where the arteries branch, or at other key areas of the artery wall damaged by high blood pressure or other factors. Interestingly, these strained or damaged sites also attract fats, particularly low-density lipoprotein (LDL) cholesterol (also known as "bad" cholesterol) that is circulating in the bloodstream.

According to mainstream medical thinking, it is the overload of these fatty substances, or lipids, in the inner wall of the artery that triggers the development of atherosclerosis. The main fatty culprit is cholesterol, most of which is either made by the liver or taken in from dietary sources, such as meat, shellfish, eggs, and other animal products.

Cholesterol plays a central role in the development of atherosclerotic plaque. This process occurs in three stages. First, it combines with proteins and another type of fat in the blood called *triglycerides* to form LDL cholesterol. This fatty complex helps cholesterol to travel through the bloodstream to other parts of the body. If too much LDL cholesterol is present, it begins to form clumps. This LDL cholesterol is sticky and tends to adhere to the interior wall of the artery, where it becomes vulnerable to damage by toxic chemicals found in the body called *free radicals* or *oxidants.* This damage by free radicals, also known as *oxidation,* then sets off an alarm in the surface endothelium layer of the artery. As part of a cascade of events, LDL cholesterol becomes oxidized or "rusted," which further increases its ability to damage the artery walls. In response, the endothelium layer sends its defensive troops into the intima. These troops involve mainly white blood cells known as *monocytes.* These immune-system cells act as scavengers, surrounding and destroying the invading LDL molecules and, in so doing, earn a new name, *macrophages.* When walls of such arteries are viewed through a microscope, accumulations of these cells are seen as yellow fatty streaks. However, these fatty streaks do not yet block the flow of blood in the lumen of the artery.

This first stage of development of atherosclerosis can begin as early as childhood and has become increasingly more common in the teenage years. One important study led by Arthur Zieske, M.D., and colleagues at Louisiana State University, found fatty streaks in the arteries of young children and advanced lesions, or plaque deposits, already developing by the teenage years. These findings refuted the long-standing belief that atherosclerosis was primarily a disease of older people.

In the second stage of plaque development, the macrophages gradually become overwhelmed by the tremendous amount of oxidized LDL they have consumed, and begin to lose their efficiency. They have become what are called *foam cells,* overstuffed with cholesterol, and begin to die. On orders from the endothelial layer of the intima, other protective changes begin to occur, such as the migration of smooth muscle cells from the middle layer (media) of the artery wall into the intima.

The soft, fatty streaks of plaque become thicker and harder as the muscle cells create fibers of protection that surround the invading foam cells. This protective layer, called the *fibrous cap,* surrounds the core of fat and overactive white blood cells. Even in this second stage where the plaque thickens significantly in the interior wall and the artery's diameter shrinks—sometimes to the point of 75 percent loss of area in the lumen—some blood still makes it to the interior of the heart muscle.

The significant difference between the first two stages of plaque development and the third stage is the formation, in this final stage, of blood clots caused by the rupture of the more fragile plaques in the artery wall. Although atherosclerosis includes an accumulation of hard, compacted plaque in the second stage, some of the advanced older plaques have thinner walls that are more brittle. These can become time bombs, particularly when there is bleeding within the plaque, and are referred to as "vulnerable" plaques. If the fragile fibrous cap ruptures, which may occur from the pressure of internal bleeding or from some other irritation in the artery, it can cause the contents of the plaque to spill into the bloodstream, thus inciting the formation of a blood clot, or thrombus, inside the artery. If this clot blocks the flow of blood in a coronary artery, it can lead to a heart attack. And once this occurs, it marks the end-stage of the atherosclerotic process, and often results in the end of one's heart and life.

CORONARY HEART DISEASE

The emergence and development of atherosclerosis in the arteries surrounding the heart is the story of coronary heart disease. When atherosclerosis takes hold in the arteries that feed the heart the nutrients and oxygen it needs to function, it puts the heart at great risk. The coronary arteries, which extend over the surface of the heart like a crown, are the channels through which these critical substances flow into the heart. (See Figure 1.1 on page 14.)

As discussed earlier, there are three main arteries that feed the entire heart: the right coronary artery, and the left anterior descending and left circumflex arteries, which branch off from the left main coronary artery. When one or more of these arteries are completely blocked, usually by swollen or ruptured plaque in the inner artery wall, the flow of oxygen to a part of the heart is cut off. This kills the cells in the area of the heart muscle that the artery feeds. When the flow of blood from a major coronary artery is not resumed within minutes, it can end with death to the heart, in other words, a fatal heart attack.

Signs and Symptoms of Coronary Heart Disease

How do you know if you have coronary heart disease? Unfortunately, this condition can be difficult to diagnose, especially in its early stages. As previously mentioned, atherosclerosis can begin to develop in childhood when fatty streaks start to line the arteries around the heart and other organs of the body. Typically, the damage progresses silently and insidiously until symptoms strike without warning in adulthood. Often, the first symptoms are a pain in the chest (angina), a heart attack (myocardial infarction), or in more severe cases, sudden cardiac death (cardiac arrest). Sudden cardiac death is the abrupt and complete loss of heart function. It accounts for 50 percent of all deaths from heart disease in the United States and other developed countries. Half of all people who die suddenly of cardiac causes have no prior symptoms of heart disease. For these people, heart disease announces itself when it is too late; they die before getting to the hospital or receiving medical care. This is the reason why doctors and healthcare practitioners emphasize early detection and, more important, prevention of heart disease.

In the remaining part of this chapter, we describe the classic symptoms of coronary heart disease and the conventional methods used by modern medicine to diagnose this condition. Coronary heart disease can be divided into two broad categories, each with a somewhat different set of symptoms, diagnostic methods, and treatments. These two categories are 1) chronic stable angina pectoris, more commonly known as *angina,* and 2) acute coronary syndromes, which include heart attacks and unstable angina, a more serious, less common form of angina that is often a precursor to a heart attack.

Angina

Angina, or angina pectoris as it is more technically called, is a type of chest pain characterized by a feeling of intense, often crushing pressure, a choking sensation, or pain that may radiate to the left arm, jaw, or back. This discomfort is usually triggered by physical exertion or emotional stress. When the exertion or stress subsides, the chest pain or discomfort is alleviated. It can also be relieved within seconds or minutes by taking nitroglycerin, a popular medicine that temporarily increases blood flow to the heart. This contrasts with unstable angina (discussed below), which may appear suddenly or occur frequently or without apparent cause, and for which the chest pain is *not* relieved by rest or nitroglycerin.

Angina pain is a sign that the heart muscle is receiving an insufficient supply of blood—a condition called *myocardial ischemia*—from coronary arteries that are severely narrowed by atherosclerosis. If you have these symptoms, most likely your doctor will recommend a stress test of your heart to diagnose the problem noninvasively.

A stress test typically involves running on a treadmill or pedaling a bicycle while your heart function and coronary blood flow are monitored using an electrocardiogram (ECG or EKG), ultrasound, or imaging device using a dye such as radioactive thallium. Another less frequently used testing method called a *pharmacologic stress test* involves the use of a drug rather than physical exercise. After the blood vessels of the heart are challenged with the drug, heart function and coronary blood flow are then monitored by one of the imaging techniques mentioned above. Both methods produce similar results.

A relatively newer method for visualizing atherosclerosis in the arteries is called *electron beam computed tomography* (EBCT). This technology is still being scientifically evaluated and compared with other noninvasive methods of heart disease diagnosis. EBCT is a type of computerized axial tomography scan (CT scan) that combines many x-ray images with the aid of a computer to generate views of the inside of the heart and coronary arteries. The scan detects calcification (calcium deposits) in the coronary arteries that have been hardened due to atherosclerosis.

If the results from one of these noninvasive tests suggest the presence of coronary heart disease, then your doctor may recommend more definitive invasive testing with coronary angiography. In this diagnostic procedure, a catheter is inserted into the heart through which radioactive dye is injected into the coronary arteries. The dye, which is visible on an x-ray, allows each of the main arteries to be viewed and the amount of narrowing, or stenosis, to be measured. Usually a vessel with more than 50 to 70 percent blockage is considered significant enough to cause symptoms of angina. Yet medical researchers are now finding that even coronary arteries narrowed by plaque growth of much smaller extent, even 20 percent, often lead to acute heart attacks. These fragile vulnerable plaques, whether they are small or large, are called *unstable atherosclerotic plaques.* Unstable plaques can rupture and cause a heart attack at almost anytime.

It is difficult to predict with conventional diagnostic methods which narrowed coronary arteries, or parts of a coronary artery, will lead to severe or life-threatening consequences later on. Although side effects of coronary angiography are not common, they can include stroke, heart attack, kidney damage, and possible death during or after the testing procedure.

Acute Coronary Syndromes

When the obstruction of a coronary artery reaches 100 percent, that is, when there is complete blockage in one of the arteries that supplies a region of the heart, then that part of the heart muscle dies. The medical term for this permanent loss of vital heart tissue is *myocardial infarction* (MI), more commonly called a *heart attack.* The consequences of a heart attack can be life threatening depending on the extent and location of the insult to the heart.

The classic symptoms of a heart attack include intense pressure, pain, tightness, or heaviness in the chest that may radiate to the neck, jaw, shoulders, arms, or back. In some people, however, a heart attack may feel like indigestion, heartburn, or nausea, and may be accompanied by vomiting. These latter symptoms occur in about half of patients with or without other symptoms. Individuals experiencing an acute heart attack may also feel short of breath, weak, dizzy, light-headed, and in extreme cases, may lose consciousness. In some cases, people have no symptoms at all; this is called a *silent* heart attack.

If a person is one of the 50 percent who make it to the hospital immediately after a heart attack, then testing with an electrocardiogram (EKG) and blood chemical tests for signs of injury to the heart muscle are used to confirm the diagnosis. In some cases, radioactive-imaging techniques and/or coronary angiography like that used for chronic stable angina are used to diagnose an acute heart attack. Unstable angina often leads to heart attack or sudden cardiac death. It is treated somewhat like a heart attack in order to relieve its unrelenting symptoms and prevent its deadly consequences.

CONCLUSION

Now that you understand a little better how the healthy cardiovascular system works, what physical changes occur as heart disease develops, and the latest medical techniques used to diagnose this condition, the question you may have is, "What can I do to prevent heart disease, or to reverse the condition if I already have it?" In the next two chapters, we'll review the approach used by conventional medicine to answer these questions by presenting the risk factors that can contribute to heart disease and by describing modern medical treatments—and their shortcomings. This will complete Section I, after which we will introduce you to natural diagnostic and therapeutic approaches that are scientific and side-effect-free and that will help you to gain total heart health!

♥ CHAPTER 2 ♥

Understanding Your Risk Factors

WHILE THE UNDERLYING CAUSES OF HEART DISEASE continue to elude modern medicine, it has identified numerous risk factors that increase your likelihood of developing the disease. Familiarizing yourself with these risk factors and their detrimental effects on the heart and arteries will give you a better grasp of the problem. This knowledge will make clear why a comprehensive, multi-modality approach to treating heart disease and its many risk factors is needed.

Conventional medicine has identified several conditions that increase your probability of developing heart disease. These conditions are called *risk factors*. While having one or more of these factors means that statistically you are at higher risk than others of developing heart disease, on the positive side, knowing which risk factors you have can help you to prevent their development.

ASSESSING YOUR RISK

Risk factors for heart disease are often grouped into two categories: modifiable risk factors and nonmodifiable risk factors. Modifiable risk factors are lifestyle-related factors over which you have control. These include high blood pressure, high cholesterol, cigarette smoking, obesity, and psychological stress. Nonmodifiable risk factors, on the other hand, are those that you cannot change. Age, gender, race and ethnicity, and heredity (family history) are considered the primary nonmodifiable factors. In recent years, these distinctions have become less important. Newer cardiovascular research indicates that with appropriate preventive strategies, you can even prevent or reverse many of the deleterious effects of nonmodifiable risk factors.

It's important to keep in mind that risk factors are not static. They are constantly interacting with one another in ways that alter your risk. If you already have coronary heart disease, for example, or if you have had a heart attack, stroke, or heart surgery, then that puts you at much higher risk for a recurrence of a heart disease–related event in the future. Also, if you have more than one risk factor, say, you have high blood pressure and diabetes, then your risk of developing heart disease becomes even higher. In many individuals, the combined effect on the coronary arteries of two risk factors is greater than the effects of the individual risk factors added together. The following sections discuss the major risk factors that are most closely linked to the development of heart disease.

High Blood Pressure

Almost 30 percent of the American population, that's one in every three adults, suffers from high blood pressure. While primarily a condition associated with aging, it is now becoming more common in young people. High blood pressure is defined as blood pressure that is greater than or equal to 140/90 mm Hg (millimeters of mercury). Another one in every three Americans has blood pressure in the "prehypertensive" range, between 120/80 and 140/90, where your blood pressure is high, but not high enough to be classified as hypertension. Although the distinction is often made between hypertension and pre-hypertension, research is finding that any increase in blood pressure higher than the normal level of 120/80 mm Hg approximately doubles your risk of heart attack, stroke, or death from heart disease. And the higher your blood pressure, the greater this risk.

The term *blood pressure* refers to the force exerted against the artery walls as blood races through them. The contractions of the heart cause a pumping action that pushes the blood through your arteries. The amount of pressure the blood exerts against the walls of the arteries depends on three factors: 1) the strength of the heart's pumping action; 2) the amount of blood coursing through the artery; and 3) the resistance created by the vessel wall. When healthy, your cardiovascular system naturally synchronizes these three factors, thereby avoiding excess pressure. It is a feat of engineering brilliance, especially when you consider that blood is pumped through thousands of miles of vessels in the body, which range from large to microscopic, and flows constantly without a breakdown or block in the flow. The elastic blood vessels are able to contract and expand as the body's needs for blood change under various circumstances. When you exercise, for example, a larger volume of blood is pumped through the system and is pumped more quickly than when you are at rest.

If, on the other hand, the blood pressure inside the arteries is elevated for a prolonged period of time, such as when you are living in a continual state of stress, it places a strain on the artery walls. Like a hose that must break or crack if too much water is pushed through it, either episodically or constantly, elevated blood pressure will eventually cause damage to the artery wall and to the artery itself, and atherosclerosis begins.

As you learned in the previous chapter, when the artery wall is injured, inflammatory and defensive responses within the artery are activated. If this injury is continuous, as it is with chronic high blood pressure, protective plaque begins to build up on the walls, creating an abnormal mass over time. These injured sites also attract fatty substances, which stimulate the healing aspect of plaque production, but which also promote further thickening of the artery. This constriction squeezes the artery, causing blood pressure to rise even higher and a vicious circle sets in. Chronic stress is considered by many physicians to be one of the primary causes of high blood pressure and is the reason why many people find their blood pressure rising over time.

Pinpointing the initial cause for prolonged high blood pressure in each person still baffles most doctors and researchers. It has been estimated that more than 95 percent of people with high blood pressure have *"essential"* or *"primary" hypertension,* meaning that the specific initial cause of their high blood pressure cannot be identified. Nevertheless, a number of lifestyle and heredity factors are thought to contribute. These include chronic psychological stress (as already mentioned), older age (half of Americans sixty years or older have hypertension), race, family background, obesity, smoking, lack of exercise, and even where you live. It is suspected that other factors such as excess consumption of alcohol and drugs and a diet high in sodium intake also contribute to essential hypertension.

The remaining 5 percent of hypertension sufferers have "secondary" hypertension, which can be attributed to an existing health problem such as kidney disease, disease of the adrenal glands, endocrine disorders, diabetes, drug-induced hypertension, and even pregnancy.

High blood pressure can have serious health consequences. Not only is it one of the main factors contributing to the buildup of atherosclerosis in the coronary arteries, where it doubles your risk of heart attack, but it also promotes the development of atherosclerosis throughout the entire circulatory system, including those areas that feed vital nutrients to the brain. In the brain, high blood pressure may cause the vessels to burst and bleed into the brain tissue, which can result in a stroke. High blood pressure can also cause kidney disease. When hypertension is combined with obesity, cigarette smoking, elevated cholesterol, or diabetes, it increases your risk of having a heart attack or a stroke several fold. The reason is that all these conditions aggravate and accelerate the atherosclerotic process.

The longest study of health in the United States, the ongoing Framingham Heart Study, has been following more than 5,000 families from Framingham,

Massachusetts, for over fifty years. As early as 1961, this study linked risk factors such as hypertension to increased risk of heart attack, stroke, and premature death.

High blood pressure can also cause heart failure, which means that the heart is not pumping enough blood out into the body. This is caused by damage to the pumping mechanism of the heart and typically results in an enlarged heart, particularly an enlarged left ventricle. In this disorder, the heart can no longer pump blood efficiently to the rest of the body. When the heart muscle is weakened or when there is damage to other organs in the body from high blood pressure, such as to the kidneys, there is an even greater probability of developing heart disease. When there is damage like this, it is called *hypertensive heart disease.*

Unfortunately, unless your blood pressure is markedly elevated, you may not know you have higher than normal blood pressure. High blood pressure frequently goes undetected until some damage has already been done, which is why it is sometimes called the *silent killer.* It's one reason why only an estimated 60 percent of people with hypertension know they have it; the other 40 percent are unaware that they have a potentially lethal medical problem. For many people, the first warning sign of high blood pressure is a heart attack.

About half of the people who know they have high blood pressure use conventional treatments to try to keep it under control. And of this one-half, only about 50 percent has it well controlled. No one is completely safe. Anyone can suffer from hypertension, even young people.

Elevated Cholesterol

As we briefly described in the previous chapter, cholesterol plays a key role in the evolution of plaque along the walls of the arteries (atherosclerosis) and in the development of coronary heart disease. When people hear the word *cholesterol,* they usually think of it as something unhealthy. While this is in part true, not all the effects of cholesterol are bad. In fact, cholesterol has an essential and beneficial role in the body.

Cholesterol is one of several fats (lipids) that are found in every body cell, including the cells in the bloodstream. The body uses cholesterol to make cell membranes, steroid and adrenal hormones, other vital substances such as bile (a substance in the intestines used for the digestion of fats), and myelin sheaths (the covering that surrounds and protects nerve cells). The liver naturally produces the majority of the cholesterol the body needs. Additional cholesterol enters the body through the foods you eat—primarily in dietary fats such as animal fats found in meat, eggs, and shellfish.

Although cholesterol is essential to your body, when too much of it builds up in your bloodstream or arteries it can become a serious problem. A high blood cholesterol level (measured in milligrams per deciliter of blood, or mg/dL) is defined as a level equal to or greater than 240 mg/dL. Because cholesterol has been shown to be the predominant substance in atherosclerotic plaque, it is now generally accepted in modern medicine as a major risk factor for the development of atherosclerosis and coronary heart disease, and a leading cause of heart attack. One of the most significant findings from the Framingham Heart Study is that the rate of heart attacks is proportionate to the level of cholesterol in the blood. Study participants who had experienced heart attacks had elevated cholesterol levels, whereas study participants with cholesterol levels of 175 mg/dL or less had very few heart attacks.

The American Heart Association estimates that nearly one in every two adults in the United States, or more than 100 million people, has elevated cholesterol levels. It is estimated that for every 1 percent increase in cholesterol, there is a 2 percent increase in the probability of a heart attack or of death from heart disease. Of the 100 million, about 40 million Americans have cholesterol levels that are so high that powerful medications are recommended to lower those levels. For the other 60 million people with elevated cholesterol, medical authorities recommend nondrug approaches alone. Yet, less than one-half of these 100 million individuals are able to adequately control their high cholesterol by conventional drug or diet approaches.

You have two main types of lipoproteins in your blood: high-density lipoprotein cholesterol (HDL) and low-density lipoprotein cholesterol (LDL). HDL cholesterol has gained a reputation for being *good* cholesterol because it acts like a clean-up crew carrying excess cholesterol out of the cells and away from the artery walls to the liver, which breaks it down and removes it from your body.

Although the purpose of LDL cholesterol is to transport cholesterol to various sites in your body for many of its cell-building functions, it is commonly referred to as harmful, or *bad* cholesterol. This is because when an excess of this cholesterol is circulating in the blood, it can attach to artery walls where it plays a leading role in the development of atherosclerosis, especially the fatty plaques that narrow the arteries and reduce blood flow. Another form of LDL cholesterol known as *very low-density lipoprotein cholesterol* (VLDL) carries more fat called *triglycerides* than LDL cholesterol. Because some VLDL cholesterol can be converted to LDL cholesterol, it is also considered to be an unhealthy type of cholesterol in large quantities.

Because of the plaque-producing role of excess LDL cholesterol and the clean-up role of HDL cholesterol, your level of risk from cholesterol is determined by calculating the ratio of HDL and LDL in your blood. To do this, your

HDL reading is subtracted from your total cholesterol reading. An HDL level less than 45 mg/dL is considered risky. A total cholesterol level of 240 mg/dL or more indicates high risk of developing heart disease. A total cholesterol reading of 200 to 239 mg/dL is considered borderline to high. About one-third of American adults are in this group. Only one-half of American adults have a normal total cholesterol level, that is, a level below 200 mg/dL.

Smoking

Many of the 4,000 chemical substances in tobacco are thought to damage health. In addition to promoting the development of cancer in the lungs and other parts of the body, as well as numerous other health problems, tobacco smoking accelerates atherosclerosis throughout the entire cardiovascular system. It has been shown to double your risk of developing heart disease.

There are many chemicals in cigarettes that contribute to atherosclerosis. Smoking is thought to directly damage the inner lining of the artery, the endothelium, which promotes the beginning of atherosclerosis. Smoking causes blood to clot more readily. Clotting combined with narrowing and hardening of the arteries can result in a blockage in a coronary artery and lead to sudden cardiac death.

If that isn't enough, nicotine in cigarette smoke stimulates the adrenal glands to secrete a hormone called *adrenaline,* which increases blood pressure and heart rate. Carbon monoxide, another highly dangerous chemical in smoke, reduces the amount of oxygen the blood can carry by attaching itself to hemoglobin (the part of red blood cells that transports oxygen throughout the body) and replacing the oxygen in your cells. Carbon monoxide also causes the arteries to constrict.

All these metabolic changes set the stage for a heart attack, especially if your arteries are already narrow from atherosclerosis. When smoking is mixed with other risk factors, their deadly effects are dramatically increased. Smokers have twice the risk of a heart attack than nonsmokers. This makes cigarette smoking a major risk factor for cardiac death. Low-tar, low-nicotine cigarettes don't completely eliminate this risk, as they still raise blood carbon monoxide levels and remain a health hazard.

Even if you do not smoke, research has revealed that inhaling secondhand smoke is harmful. Being in the presence of cigarette smoke has been found to promote heart disease.

Because smoking is not only highly dangerous but also addictive, one of the big challenges within the medical community is how to help people quit this habit. The latest statistics show that more than 20 percent of the American population smokes. Of the 400,000 people who die a year from smoking-related causes, most die from heart attacks, not lung cancer. And 40,000 individuals a year die from secondhand-smoke-related causes. Unfortunately, recent surveys show increases in tobacco use among teenagers and women in the United States.

Diabetes

In the past decade, the rate of diabetes has increased 50 percent in the American population. This is likely attributable to the alarming increase in obesity among adults and children (see the next section, "Obesity"). In diabetes, too much blood sugar (glucose) collects in the bloodstream rather than being stored inside the cells throughout the body. A clinical diagnosis of diabetes is indicated when fasting blood sugar levels are higher than 126 mg/dL (measured in milligrams of glucose in one-tenth liter of blood). Diabetes does not result from eating a lot of sugar that collects in the blood. Rather, it is a failure of the cells of the body to sequester and properly metabolize and assimilate the sugar that is produced or ingested. Normally, the body converts some of the food you eat into glucose, which provides energy for your cells. This glucose is distributed throughout your body by the bloodstream. A hormone called *insulin* allows the glucose to enter your cells.

In individuals with diabetes, there is a deficiency in insulin-stimulated storage of glucose by the cells of the body. In type 1 diabetes, sometimes called *juvenile-onset diabetes* because it typically begins in childhood, the pancreas is unable to make enough insulin to cause transport of glucose into the cells. In type 2 diabetes, formerly called *adult-onset diabetes,* the cells of the body are not able to respond to the insulin the pancreas does produce, and far too much glucose remains in the bloodstream.

Approximately 20 million Americans have been diagnosed with diabetes and of them, 95 percent have type 2. It has been estimated that an additional 5 million Americans have type 2 diabetes but are unaware they have the disease. Type 2 diabetes has increased at an alarming rate worldwide over the past decade, affecting not only adults, for whom it was originally named, but now children as well. Type 1 diabetes is also on the rise and is estimated to affect 1.5 million young Americans.

If you have diabetes, your risk for cardiovascular disease is significantly higher. The probability of dying from a heart attack is four to seven times greater for someone with diabetes than for a healthy person. An elevated blood sugar level, even without a clinical diagnosis of diabetes, is considered a strong predictor of heart disease. There are several reasons for this. First, high levels of sugar in the bloodstream damage blood vessels and stimulate the development of atherosclerosis. Second, people with high blood sugar levels also tend to have a higher fat content, such as triglycerides and cholesterol, in their blood, which, as we have seen, plays a key role in the development of atherosclerosis. These factors dramatically reduce the ability of your heart and other organs to get the vital nutrients and oxygen they need to do their work.

According to the American Heart Association, 75 percent of all diabetes sufferers die from heart attacks. Some studies suggest that even if you have borderline high blood sugar (fasting blood glucose of 110–125 mg/dL), a condition that is called *impaired glucose tolerance* or *prediabetes,* you have a similar risk as those that have been diagnosed with diabetes. More than one in six Americans has diabetes or a precursor to this condition.

While modern medicine does not understand the exact causes of type 2 diabetes, a sedentary lifestyle, an unhealthy diet, and obesity are suspected of being major contributing factors to this burgeoning epidemic.

Obesity

If you are an American, you may likely be among the 60 percent of the population that is overweight. Overweight Americans abound, with 30 percent of these people classified as obese. What's even more disturbing is that obesity among children is rapidly increasing. Today, more than 25 percent of children in America are considered obese. These figures are very bad news for Americans since even being 20 percent above your ideal weight more than doubles your risk of heart disease. Larger weight gains mean even higher chances of developing heart problems. This makes excess weight a major risk factor for heart disease.

The American Heart Association admits that some reasons for this higher risk are unclear, but others are not. An excess of body weight has been found to raise LDL cholesterol and triglyceride levels, lower protective HDL cholesterol levels, increase blood pressure, and promote type 2 diabetes, all conditions that have been found to significantly contribute to the development of atherosclerosis.

Rather than rely on a bathroom scale to measure whether you are overweight, doctors and healthcare practitioners often use a more reliable method called the *body mass index* (BMI). The BMI measures the body's composition by calculating the percentage of body weight that is fat. This calculation is determined by comparing how much a person weighs to how tall he or she is. This is done by referring to a special BMI chart found in most medical offices, or you can calculate your own by referring to any number of online BMI calculators (for example, the National Heart, Lung, and Blood Institute's BMI calculator, which can be found on their website: http://nhlbisupport.com/bmi/bmicalc.htm). According to current federal weight guidelines, a person is considered to be overweight if they have a BMI of 25 to 29; obese, if the BMI is 30 or more; and morbidly obese if the BMI is 40 or greater.

Another indicator of heart disease risk is where most of your fat is located. If you tend to have an apple shape, meaning that you have a big belly, you are at more risk for coronary heart disease, as well as high blood pressure, diabetes, stroke, and certain types of cancer than if you are pear shaped, where more of your fat is around your hips and thighs. Research has shown that when there is increased abdominal body fat, there is a greater tendency for this fat to break down and accumulate in the arteries.

Another way of telling whether you are carrying too much weight around the middle is to measure your waist at its narrowest point and to compare that with your hips. To measure your hips, determine the circumference just above the highest point of your hips, that is, at their widest. Then compare these two measurements by dividing the waist measurement by the hip measurement. For example, if your waist measures 29 inches and your hips are 38 inches, divide 29 by 38 and you get a ratio of 0.76 to 1. This is considered within a healthy range. If the ratio is less than 0.8 to 1 for women and less than 0.95 to 1 for men, it is considered healthy. Some studies have suggested that a waistline of more than 35 inches for women and 40 inches for men are also indicators of higher risk for heart disease.

Overweight people who are at high risk for heart disease are advised to lose weight toward ideal BMI and waist circumference. Americans spend billions on weight control and exercise programs to do this. Some are successful, but many are not. Two-thirds of those who lose weight gain it back within five years.

Sedentary Lifestyle

Physical inactivity and a sedentary lifestyle have become hallmarks of the American lifestyle. Recent research estimates that inactivity increases your risk of heart disease by 50 percent. Despite these odds, 60 percent of American adults do less than the daily minimum level of exercise recommended. Worse yet, nearly 25 percent are totally inactive.

You are considered sedentary, if:

• You sit most of the day.

• You hardly ever walk more than a block.

• Your leisure activities don't involve physical movement.

• You are physically inactive in your job.

• You get less than twenty to thirty minutes of exercise most days of the week.

Physical activity plays an essential role in the optimum health of the body, including the health of the heart and lungs. While most recommendations suggest a minimum of twenty to thirty minutes of physical activity on most, if not all, days of the week, even a moderate increase in activity can help reduce the risk of heart disease. Research shows that regular physical activity promotes weight loss, cuts your risk of glucose intolerance and type 2 diabetes by lowering blood sugar, reduces high blood pressure and total cholesterol, improves circulation, and relieves stress. Obviously, this has a positive effect on the health of your coronary arteries too. But, even though most of us know how beneficial exercise is, too many of us do not actually make time to exercise regularly.

Stress

Given the fast-paced, high-pressured lives of people today, it's not surprising that almost everyone suffers from some form of chronic stress. Large population surveys conducted by scientists affiliated with the National Institute for Mental Health (NIMH) have found that one in ten Americans suffers from an anxiety-related disorder. The surveys also showed that nearly one in ten people is depressed. Anxiety and depression are two of the most common manifestations of stress.

Stress is one risk that is not limited to the American lifestyle. Researchers at the World Health Organization (WHO, the United Nation's agency for tracking health worldwide) have observed that depression is becoming a global epidemic and coincides with the epidemic of heart disease prevalent in modern urbanized societies. Cardiology research over the past forty years, including studies that our colleagues and we have conducted at the Institute for Natural Medicine and Prevention, have found that in addition to anxiety and depression a variety of negative emotional states such as anger, hostility, low self-esteem, and social isolation can cascade into a range of physical health problems. In fact, all types of stresses—psychological, emotional, and social—greatly increase your risk for hypertension and heart disease.

High stress levels may seem common to modern life, but it may surprise you to learn that the effects of psychological stress on health have been researched by conventional medicine for centuries. This association dates back to the ancient Greek physician Hippocrates, who is considered the father of modern medicine, and more recently to the well-known nineteenth-century physician Sir William Osler, who stated, "Mental worry, severe grief, or sudden shock may precede directly the onset of the attack of anginal chest pain."

Two of the earliest researchers in the twentieth century to study the effects of stress on the cardiovascular system were cardiologists Meyer Friedman, M.D., and Ray Rosenman, M.D. Their initial research led to their discovery that some people exhibit stronger reactions to stress than other people, which makes them more susceptible to heart disease. This and subsequent research spawned the idea of the *Type A behavior pattern*, a term coined in 1964.

Individuals with Type A behavior tend to be hard driving; they strive for perfection and feel constantly pressured by deadlines and tasks to accomplish. They also tend to be highly competitive and typically overcommitted to their work, trying to accomplish more and more in less and less time. As a result, work and personal relationships suffer; they become irritable, easily frustrated, and impatient or critical of others, and sometimes even hostile. Many people in America and other developed countries share the qualities of the Type A behavior pattern. And while some of these characteristics may have served as catalysts for many great accomplishments, this type of behavior eventually takes its toll on the body.

Building on the early findings of Friedman and Rosenman, researchers began to contrast the Type A style with other types of personalities. From this, the concept of the Type B behavior pattern was conceived. Researchers observed that those who exhibited a Type B pattern were still interested in achievement, but they were more relaxed, less hurried, and more accepting of their pace and of the people with whom they interacted. Studies in 1960s, 1970s, and early 1980s documented that people with the Type A behavior pattern are twice as likely to develop heart disease than are people with Type B personalities.

Since the 1980s, research has identified more specific emotional states to watch out for: feeling chronically hostile, depressed, anxious, or angry significantly heightens the risk for coronary heart disease. Low self-esteem, low sense of social support, stress on the job or at home, and poor capacity to cope with stressful situations increase the risk as well.

A lead article in the March 2005 issue of the *Journal of the American College of Cardiology* reviewed two decades of research showing that stress significantly contributes to the development of heart disease. The review by Alan Rozanski, M.D., and colleagues explained that these psychosocial factors contribute to the development of heart disease in three ways: they directly contribute to the development of atherosclerosis; they promote unhealthy lifestyle habits such as smoking, excessive alcohol consumption, inactivity, and poor diet, which also damage the cardiovascular system; and they provide barriers to successful change in unhealthy lifestyles after disease has set in.

When you are constantly reacting to stressful events, your sympathetic nervous system remains on high alert. The sympathetic nervous system is one of two divisions of the autonomic nervous system responsible for preparing the body to cope with threatening situations. Stress causes this system to release large amounts of adrenaline and noradrenaline from the nervous system and adrenal glands into the bloodstream. These two stress hormones speed up the body's metabolic rate, and increase alertness and energy, which in turn cause the arteries to constrict and the heart rate to increase in order to pump more blood. These protective mechanisms are part of what is called the body's *fight or flight response*. While they are critical in the face of an immediate threat, if these mechanisms are chronically activated, they can result in high blood pressure and high heart reactivity, which damage the walls of the arteries. And, as we know, this damage precipitates the development of atherosclerosis, the source of heart disease.

When you are threatened, the adrenal glands also release copious amounts of another major stress hormone, cortisol. Like adrenaline and noradrenaline, this hormone helps to prepare the body to perform rapidly in emergencies. However, if excessive amounts of cortisol continue to circulate in the bloodstream because of chronic stress, they can cause damage to the walls of the arteries and accelerate the development of atherosclerosis and heart disease. Higher-than-normal levels of these stress hormones over the long-term put you at great risk not only for high blood pressure and atherosclerosis, but also for thrombosis (blood clotting at the site of an atherosclerosis plaque) and arrhythmias (irregular rhythm of the heart), both of which can lead to sudden cardiac death. To make matters worse, chronic stress promotes other risk factors of heart disease, such as obesity, high cholesterol, smoking, excessive alcohol consumption, and physical inactivity. Very few people, if any, are immune from the psychological stresses and strains of modern society. This puts virtually everyone at risk for stress-related heart disease.

Excessive Alcohol Consumption

Drinking alcohol in excess is also associated with higher rates of heart disease. Studies have shown that an excessive intake of alcohol—more than two drinks a day for men or one drink per day for women—raises blood pressure and significantly increases your risk for atherosclerosis and heart disease by damaging the inside of the blood vessels. Some individuals, particularly women, may be more sensitive to the adverse effects of alcohol on the heart, possibly due to less body weight or other factors.

In addition, consuming too much alcohol can lead to depression; it impairs the functioning of your brain cells and disturbs diet and other healthy lifestyle behaviors. Moreover, alcohol is full of empty calories and easily turns into fat and unwanted weight.

Aging

Aging is another factor associated with increased rates of heart disease. As people age, there is a tendency for their blood pressure to increase steadily with each year of life. Interestingly, in traditional, nonurbanized societies, where people's daily routines more closely follow nature's rhythms, blood pressure does not increase with age, and diseases of the heart are relatively rare. These societies offer modern medicine a lesson on the promotion of heart health. In modernized societies, however, the rates of heart disease for men and women increase threefold from about age thirty-five to eight-five. This is likely related to our modern lifestyle with its attendant stresses and strains and unhealthy behaviors.

Gender

Women tend to develop coronary heart disease on average about ten years later than men. Men have higher rates of heart disease than women until about age fifty or fifty-five. As such, heart disease has traditionally been thought of as a "man's disease." However, nothing could be farther from the truth. After menopause, a woman's risk of heart disease increases dramatically. At this point, heart disease strikes men and women at equal rates. By age sixty, heart disease is the leading cause of death in women.

According to the American Heart Association, 250,000 women die every year of heart disease. Other figures show that women suffer one-half of all fatal heart attacks. These statistics make heart disease the number-one cause of death in women, taking five times more lives every year than breast cancer.

Women with heart disease may exhibit different symptoms than men, and because of this the disease is more often underdiagnosed. Moreover, the development of atherosclerosis is likely to be slowed down or sped up by a person's hormonal state. For example, the decreased amount of estrogen circulating in a woman's bloodstream after menopause may cause changes in cholesterol (increased LDL, reduced HDL) and increased glucose intolerance. Unfortunately, simple replacement of sex hormones—administering estrogen as a drug—is not the answer that modern medicine once thought it was. Recent results from the Women's Health Initiative study of more than 16,000 post-menopausal women found that women who were given hormone replacement therapy with estrogen and progesterone had *increased* rates of heart attack, stroke, and breast cancer compared with women who did not receive hormone therapy. For these reasons, medical authorities no longer recommend hormone therapy for prevention of heart disease in women. Later in Section II, we'll recommend some natural approaches for prevention of heart disease in women, as well as men. These recommendations have been shown through scientific research and extensive clinical experience to be without harmful side effects and to promote mind-body health in a holistic way.

Race and Ethnic Background

Race and ethnicity are implicated as risk factors for heart disease and high blood pressure. For example, African Americans are more likely to develop hypertension and to have a more severe form of it than white Americans; they are also 50 percent more likely to die from heart disease than white Americans. Hispanic Americans experience about double the rate of diabetes as white Americans.

It has been suggested that many of these differences are not attributable to race or ethnicity per se, but rather to environmental stresses created by poor living conditions, low socioeconomic and education levels, as well as many other psychological stresses associated with minority social and lifestyle conditions. One example that calls into question the role of ethnicity as a risk factor for heart disease is the effect of living in westernized society on Japanese people. Native Asian people living in Japan have relatively low rates of heart disease. However, Japanese people living in California and following a western lifestyle have much higher rates of heart disease than their counterparts in their native country. Likewise, Japanese men and women living in Hawaii, geographically midway between Japan and the United States, have heart disease rates that are halfway between those that live on the U.S. mainland and in Japan. These data suggest that lifestyle according to the traditional ways of life in Japan, even in recent decades, contribute to lower rates of heart disease compared with the American lifestyle.

Family History of Heart Disease

If your parents or siblings had heart disease before age fifty-five (for a father or brother) or age sixty-five (for a mother or sister), you are 30 to 50 percent more likely to develop early heart disease yourself. Some people have a genetic predisposition for very high cholesterol levels called *familial hypercholesterolemia,* which adds to the risk. Other genetic propensities that are commonly found in families are the tendency for high blood pressure, moderately high cholesterol, diabetes, and obesity, all of which predispose you to heart disease.

As pointed out earlier, the role of nonmodifiable factors such as preprogrammed genes in heart disease is considered by many medical experts to be much less than previously thought. One reason, it was later realized, is that children who share their genes with their parents also share their environments, living conditions, and lifestyle patterns with their parents. Findings from studies of migrants also suggest that while genetic makeup plays a role, it is only one of many contributors. Many scientists now believe that your environment and lifestyle play a stronger role in determining your risk of developing heart disease than your genes.

CONCLUSION

In this chapter, we reviewed modern medicine's understanding of the major risk factors that predispose you to heart disease and its life-threatening consequences. This rapid-fire review is a reminder that if you presently have one or more of these risk factors, then you are probably in the early stages of heart disease and are well on your way to the damaging effects that take the lives of so many people in the world. Despite the progress that conventional medicine has made in helping people reduce or control some of these risk factors in their lives, millions continue to suffer from heart disease each year. This is because medical science's knowledge, diagnosis, and treatment of this disease are still incomplete.

There needs to be a deeper understanding of the core causes of heart disease if we are to truly understand how to prevent or reverse it. Fortunately, there is a comprehensive, natural system for gaining total heart health that has been scientifically verified and successfully used by millions of people. But before we present this program in detail, the next chapter will discuss the methods presently used by conventional medicine in its efforts to manage heart disease, and the reasons why they fall short of the goal of total heart health.

CHAPTER 3

Modern Heart Medicine and Its Limitations

MODERN MEDICINE HAS ATTEMPTED TO PREVENT and treat heart disease and its risk factors for the last fifty years. These efforts have included aware-ness campaigns, extensive drug therapies, and high-tech diagnostic and surgical methods. More than $300 billion is spent on the diagnosis and treatment of heart disease each year. Yet, despite these modern advances, heart disease continues to take more than 1 million lives in the United States each year, and over 17 million lives per year worldwide. Less than a century ago, the proportion of people who died of heart disease was about one in five. Today, this number has risen to almost one in two. Even more disconcerting, the hazardous side effects of modern medicine itself takes the lives of more than 250,000 people per year, making it the third leading cause of death after heart disease and stroke. This is not a winning battle.

This chapter presents an overview of the major medications and sur-gical procedures used by the medical community in its effort to control the damaging and life-threatening effects of heart disease. In doing so, the inadequacies in the conventional approaches to heart disease will be discussed. It will begin to make sense that to obtain total heart health, you need to go beyond treating the symptoms of heart disease, as mod-ern medicine does, and treat the ultimate causes of heart disease.

Conventional methods for preventing heart disease generally fall under the categories of primary and secondary prevention. Primary prevention involves interventions that are used *before* you have cardiovascular dis-ease. The focus during this stage is on risk-factor control, often through the use of drugs and lifestyle modifications. Secondary prevention involves interventions that are used after a person is already diagnosed with cardiovascular disease. This is usually called *treatment* rather than *prevention,* but its goal is to prevent the disease from getting worse and doing even more damage. Secondary prevention commonly includes drugs and surgical interventions. In the following sections, we discuss some of the pros and cons of common drugs and surgical procedures used in the conventional prevention and treatment of heart disease.

DRUGS

Various medications are commonly prescribed for the treatment of risk factors and symptoms of heart disease. They are used both as primary and secondary prevention. The most common of these drugs are discussed below.

Diuretics

Diuretics, or "water pills," are a class of drugs commonly used to treat high blood pressure. Diuretics dilate the blood vessels and decrease the volume of blood flowing through them. They are able to reduce blood volume by blocking the kidney's ability to absorb salt. This causes a flushing of salt and water out into the urine. This works because salt plays an important role in keeping water in the body: where salt goes, water goes. Less water in the body means less water in the bloodstream, and hence less blood volume circulating in the body. When the volume is lower, the pressure against the artery walls is lower and blood flows more easily. With more space for the blood to flow, the heart doesn't have to work as hard to push the blood through. The result is a decrease in blood pressure.

The group of diuretics most commonly used to treat high blood pressure are the thiazides, and combination products that contain thiazides. Examples of the most frequently used diuretics include chlorthalidone (Hygroton), hydrochlorothiazide (Hydrodiurel, Esidrix), hydrochlorothiazide plus amiloride (Moduretic), hydrochlorothiazide plus spironolactone (Aldactazide), hydrochlorothiazide plus triamterene (Dyazide, Maxide), indapamide (Lozol), and metolazone (Zaroxolyn).

Diuretics are considered a cornerstone in the treatment of high blood pressure. They are able to lower arterial pressure in a few days, and are often combined with other drugs to enhance their ability to control blood pressure. Most people with hypertension have to use more than one medicine to bring their blood pressure down. In fact, fewer than half the people with high blood pressure can control it with only a single type of drug. One-third of hypertensive patients need three or more different medicines. For example, people often receive prescriptions for use of diuretics along with ACE inhibitors and beta-blockers (discussed later in this section), as the add-on drugs may enhance the effectiveness of diuretic drugs.

Diuretics have received the most use and the most research regarding their effect on high blood pressure, even though research has shown that taking them for an extended time increases your risk for some damaging side effects. One concern is that along with the expelling of salt and water is the significant excretion of other important minerals, such as potassium and magnesium, both of which are critical for the healthy functioning of the heart. It has been found that significant loss of these two electrolytes can predispose you to an irregular heartbeat and sudden cardiac death.

Other side effects of long-term use of diuretics that you may experience are elevated levels of blood sugar, cholesterol, and triglycerides. Diuretics can also cause too much acid and salt to build up in your bloodstream and joints. This can lead to gouty arthritis, which is painful and can damage your joints. Dangerously low blood pressure and depression are also a risk when you take these drugs. Other common problems are stomach upset and cold hands and feet, which affects one in ten diuretic users.

Diuretics may cause impotency. Men who receive long-term treatment often develop erectile dysfunction, even more so than with the other drugs used for treating high blood pressure. This side effect has been found to go away as soon as the diuretics are stopped.

Beta-blockers

Beta-blockers are a frequently prescribed class of drugs that are used to treat high blood pressure, angina, congestive heart failure, and arrhythmia, and for people who have had a heart attack. Beta-blockers reduce pressure in the blood vessels by reducing the constriction of the arteries and by decreasing the rate and volume of blood being pumped by your heart.

As discussed earlier, when you are highly stressed or active, your sympathetic nervous system becomes more active. This causes the nerves surrounding the heart to stimulate the release of stress hormones such as noradrenaline. As a result, the arteries constrict and the heart beats faster so your body can quickly respond to threats and other intense or emergency-like situations. This causes greater pressure in the arteries, and as we know, if this pressure is prolonged, then problems related to chronically high blood pressure arise. Beta-blockers block the ability of the receptors of the heart to respond to noradrenaline, thereby causing the arteries to relax (dilate) and the heart to beat slower and less forcefully.

During highly active or stressful times, the sympathetic nervous system also stimulates the release of the hormone renin by your kidneys. This hormone causes the kidneys to retain salt and water. As a result, water enters the bloodstream and increases the volume of blood flowing through the arteries. This also increases the pressure in the arteries. Beta-blockers help reduce this pressure by blocking the release of renin. With less renin, the body gets rid of salt and water and the volume of blood decreases.

When the arteries become more relaxed and the rate and the volume of blood being pumped through the blood vessels is reduced through the use of beta-blockers, the pressure in the arteries is also reduced. This lowers your blood pressure readings and eases the workload on your heart. If you have had a heart attack, it is thought that beta-blockers can help prevent a second attack. The following beta-blockers are commonly prescribed for this purpose: atenolol (Tenormin), carvediolol (Coreg), labetalol (Normodyne, Trandate), metoprolol (Lopressor, Toprol XL), nadolol (Corgard), pindolol (Visken), propanolol (Inderal), and timolol (Blocadren).

Beta-blockers can be hard on your body, including the heart. They cause abnormal slowing of the heartbeat and impair circulation. One effect of this is cold hands and feet. Beta-blockers can also cause depression, fatigue, weakness, lightheadedness, and insomnia. A common complaint is reduced libido, and they have been found to cause sexual dysfunction, especially in men. They impair the functioning of the lungs, including the constriction of the bronchi, and have been known to precipitate bronchitis and asthma attacks, wheezing, and breathlessness. They have been found to mask the symptoms of low blood sugar and create potentially serious complications in people with diabetes.

Beta-blockers have also been known to raise triglyceride levels and reduce HDL cholesterol, which is particularly hazardous if you already have heart disease. Also of great concern is that this type of drug may weaken the pumping strength of the heart and cause heart failure in some individuals. These side effects are serious. Your physician should closely monitor any change in the use of these drugs. Abrupt termination of their use can cause severe angina and even a heart attack.

Angiotensin-Converting Enzyme Inhibitors (ACE Inhibitors)

Angiotensin-converting enzyme inhibitors are newer than many of the cardio-vascular drugs used by conventional medicine. They are prescribed as a frontline drug for treating high blood pressure and congestive heart failure, and for reducing the risk of heart attack. They received their name because they prevent the angiotensin-converting enzyme (ACE) from converting the hormone angiotensin I into a modified and more active form of the hormone, called *angiotensin II.*

Angiotensin I is responsible for regulating the amount of blood circulating through the body. The body activates this hormone when it detects an insufficient flow of blood. Angiotensin I then stimulates the body to retain salt and water so that there will be greater blood volume, and it causes the blood vessels to constrict in an effort to push more blood quickly through the blood-stream. This is one of your body's key mechanisms for regulation of your cardiovascular system, as it allows the cells in the body to be supplied with the increased nutrients and oxygen it needs when quickly moving from lesser to greater activity.

The trouble begins when your body detects a greater need for blood because it craves more oxygen and nutrients for prolonged periods, as in atherosclerosis or chronic stress. ACE then converts angiotensin I into angiotensin II, which constricts the blood vessels. The result is higher blood pressure.

By blocking ACE with ACE inhibitors, the arteries relax, blood pressure decreases, and demands on the heart decrease. There are many ACE inhibitors. Some common ones are benazepril (Lotensin), captopril (Capoten), enalapril (Vasotec), fosinopril (Monopril), lisinopril (Zestril, Prinivil), moexipril (Univasc), ramipril (Altace), and trandolapril (Mavik).

As with all modern medicines, ACE inhibitors come with their own set of side effects. One particularly annoying problem resulting from the use of these drugs is a persistent dry cough, thought to be caused by the continued production by the body of chemicals called *peptides,* which dilate your arteries but are also thought to trigger contractions of the small tubes in your lungs called *bronchioles.* This happens in up to one-third of people taking ACE inhibitors, and some people switch over to another drug because of it.

ACE inhibitors may also cause skin rashes, stomach disorders, reduced appetite, and loss of taste. They sometimes lower blood pressure too quickly or can cause persistent low blood pressure. This can make you feel faint when you are active, or when increasing your activity, such as getting up quickly after sitting. This is why physicians often suggest that the dose of the drug be increased *gradually.* Initial use of an ACE inhibitor can cause greater dizziness and may require taking it at bedtime.

Another potentially serious side effect with ACE inhibitors is that high levels of potassium can accumulate in the blood. If not detected and modified, this can cause nausea, diarrhea and, if severe, an arrhythmia (irregular or fast beating of the heart), which can lead to sudden death due to a heart attack.

There is also the possibility of kidney damage. Studies show that these drugs may reduce the ability of the kidneys to get rid of waste products. In people with preexisting kidney disease, these drugs may cause excessively low blood pressure and acute kidney failure.

Angiotensin II Receptor Blockers (ARBs)

The effects of ARBs in the body are similar to the effects of ACE inhibitors in that they also prevent angiotensin II from causing the blood vessels to constrict and blood volume to increase. However, instead of blocking the formation of angiotensin II from angiotensin I, as in the case of ACE inhibitors, angiotensin II receptor blockers prevent angiotensin II that has already been made from binding to its receptors in the blood vessels. They prevent its action rather than its formation. Angiotensin II receptor blockers have a similar effect on lowering blood pressure as do ACE Inhibitors. Examples of commonly used ARBs include losartan (Cozaar), losartan and hydrochlorothiazide (Hyzaar), and valsartan (Diovan).

Being a newer class of drug, long-term effects from taking ARBs are less well known at this time. They have risks similar to ACE inhibitors in that they may cause very low blood pressure and kidney failure in people who have kidney disease. They can also greatly raise potassium levels in the body, which can cause nausea, diarrhea, or arrhythmia, leading to sudden death due to a heart attack. On the other hand, ARBs are sometimes preferable to ACE inhibitors because they do not cause cough or rash as often as ACE inhibitors.

Calcium Channel Blockers

Calcium channel blockers are a class of drugs prescribed for angina, high blood pressure, and arrhythmia. They inhibit the entry of calcium atoms into the muscle cells of the heart and arteries. Throughout your daily activities, the muscles of your heart and arteries expand and contract, which allows them to do the work of pumping blood. To help these muscles contract, calcium atoms flow through tiny calcium channels located in the membranes of muscle cells. This contraction causes the arteries to constrict. As a result, blood pressure in the arteries increases. If your muscles are constantly constricting due to ongoing stressful activity, or if your arteries are already atherosclerotic, this can become a problem leading to, or exacerbating, heart disease.

Calcium channel blockers work as their name suggests by blocking calcium from going through the calcium channels, so the muscles contract less strongly. This helps the heart muscle relax, causing it to pump less blood to the body and to need less oxygen. The muscles of the arteries also relax, which allows the blood to flow through more easily, making the heart's job easier. This lowers your blood pressure and helps prevent heart failure.

The following are some of the most frequently prescribed calcium channel blockers: amlodipine (Norvasc), diltiazem (Cardizem, Dilacor), felodipine (Plendil), nicardipine (Cardene), nifedipine (Adalat, Procardia), and verapamil (Calan, Isoptin, Verelan).

Side effects from the use of calcium channel blockers can vary depending on which type is used. Side effects may include headaches, flushing (redness in the face), and rash. Swollen ankles have also been reported.

Most calcium channel blockers cause excessive lowering of blood pressure, while some have caused excessive slowing of the heartbeat. In addition, abnormally fast, slow, or uneven heartbeat has resulted from the use of these drugs. Studies have linked them to an increased risk of heart attack and congestive heart failure. For people who have had heart failure after a heart attack, calcium channel blockers have been found to make the symptoms worse, and in some cases, to have caused death.

Alpha Receptor Blockers

This class of drugs blocks noradrenaline receptors in blood vessels from responding to noradrenaline and causes them to dilate. This causes blood pressure to go down. Members of this class of drug include doxazosin (Cardura), prazosin (Minipress), and terazosin (Hytrin).

Side effects are relatively common and include low blood pressure and fainting. Possible side effects of long-term use include irregular or skipped heartbeats, headache, and nervousness.

Vasodilators

These agents relax smooth muscle in the arteries and lower blood pressure. They are usually given with diuretics because vasodilators can cause fluid retention and swelling. The most common vasodilator drugs include hydralazine (Apresoline) and minoxidil (Loniten).

Hydralazine frequently causes digestive disturbances and an immune disease—drug-induced lupus syndrome—in which the body's white blood cells attack its own tissues. Minoxidil causes excessive hair growth.

Statins

Statins are the most popular and most heavily promoted type of drug for lowering levels of cholesterol in the blood. They work by interfering with the body's production of LDL cholesterol. As you may remember, cholesterol is produced by the liver to be used in your body for several different functions, including the formation of cells. But when too much cholesterol, particularly LDL cholesterol, accumulates in the blood through ingestion of dietary fats or excess production by the liver, the body can't dispose of it effectively and hardening and thickening of the arteries results.

Statins help reduce the amount of cholesterol in the body by blocking the liver from making it. Statin drugs do this by interfering with the enzyme called *HMG-CoA reductase* that tells the liver to make more cholesterol. As a result, the cholesterol levels in your blood falls. When this happens, the liver also takes up more cholesterol from the blood to store it for future needs. This leads to a reduction of LDL cholesterol in the bloodstream.

Statins have been found to reduce the risk of heart attack. For people who have heart disease, it has been thought to reduce their chances of dying in the next five years by nearly one-third. However, as pointed out by Peter Wiley, M.D., Chief of Cardiology at Brigham and Women's Hospital of Harvard Medical School, even with statin therapy, "most events still happen." This means that even when one-third of events are reduced, two-thirds of cardiac deaths and heart attacks still occur in individuals at risk. Some research has also shown that if you have had bypass surgery and take statins, you are less likely to need a repeat operation. Statins have been found to lower triglyceride levels as well.

There are many statins on the market. Some of the most prescribed are atorvastatin (Lipitor), fluvastatin (Lescol), lovastatin (Mevacor), pravastatin (Pravachol), rosuvastatin (Crestor), and simvastatin (Zocor).

Although the medical community promotes statins strongly because of their cholesterol-lowering capability, the number of side effects associated with their use expands with further testing and with more time. Some of these potential side effects include headaches, upset stomachs, rashes, blurred vision, fatigue, and insomnia.

One side effect that is of particular concern is the effect of statins on the liver. In some people, statins seem to cause liver toxicity and liver problems. Some research implies that taking statins puts you at risk for liver damage and eventual liver failure. Muscle inflammation, weakness, pain, and damage have also been found, although these may not be as common. More recent research implicates statins as a cause of heart failure. Because statins are relatively new and have not been tested for more than six years, it is not really known just how dangerous they are when taken over longer periods of time.

Resins

Resins, which are also known as *bile acid sequestrants,* belong to an older group of drugs that is prescribed for lowering cholesterol and other lipids such as triglycerides in the blood. Resins reduce cholesterol by binding to the bile acids in the intestines and blocking their reabsorption into the body. Bile is a greenish-brown fluid that is produced in the liver from cholesterol. This bile is released in the intestines to help with digestion and the absorption of fat into the body.

When resins bind to the bile in the intestines, they prevent the bile from being absorbed. Instead, it is excreted. And because bile is made from cholesterol, this means cholesterol is also excreted. Also, because the bile goes out of the body with the resins, the liver has to make more bile for the body to use. The result of this is more cholesterol being taken out of the blood to make the bile. This causes your cholesterol level to fall.

Colestipol (Colestid) and colesevelam (Welchol) are examples of this type of drug. Some of the possible side effects caused by resins are constipation and other stomach and intestinal problems such as flatulence, nausea, and vomiting. Another major drawback to resins is that they can reduce the absorption of fat-soluble nutrients the body needs such as vitamins A, D, E, and K. This can cause many problems in the body. For example, with reduced long-term absorption of vitamins A and K, bleeding disorders and visual impairment may be experienced.

Fibrates

Although fibrates have some effect on lowering LDL and raising HDL cholesterol levels, they are mainly prescribed for people with excessive triglyceride levels. Fibrates are thought to reduce this blood fat by stimulating the action of an enzyme called *lipoprotein lipase.* The normal role of lipoprotein lipase in the liver is to break down the triglycerides in the blood. This allows the triglycerides to be used for energy by the muscles, with any excess being stored in the tissues under the surface of the skin for later use.

Fibrates stimulate the action of lipoprotein lipase, thereby making the enzyme break down more of the triglycerides in the blood. This reduces the amount of triglycerides in the bloodstream, and deposits and uses them elsewhere in the body. Fenofibrate (Tricor) and gemfibrozil (Lopid) are the most commonly used fibrates.

The problems associated with fibrates are similar to those associated with statins and other lipid-lowering drugs. With their unnatural involvement with the liver, the energy system of the muscles, and the storage of excess fatty substances in the body, it is not unexpected that there would be problems in these areas.

Fibrates have been found to cause nausea, diarrhea, and weight gain. The World Health Organization (WHO) and the *Physicians' Desk Reference* also cite research showing a higher probability of deaths due to gall bladder disease, cancer, and pancreatitis resulting from the use of this class of drugs. In addition, these drugs may damage the liver.

Taking fibrates has also been linked to muscle pain and damage to the muscles. This is especially the case when they are taken with statins. If you are taking fibrates, have the level of creatine kinase in your blood checked regularly, as this enzyme is found in the blood when muscles break down. Also, there have been rare cases where the damage to muscle tissue causes a malfunction in the kidneys.

Niacin

The B vitamin niacin, also called *nicotinic acid,* was one of the first agents used to lower cholesterol. When used in mega doses, this vitamin was found to lower

LDL cholesterol and triglycerides by interfering with their production in the body. It also increases HDL cholesterol. (The doses required for niacin's effects on cholesterol are many times higher than the recommended daily requirement for this vitamin.)

In one study, taking 6 milligrams of niacin a day was found to reduce LDL cholesterol by 10 percent and triglycerides by 26 percent. In the same study, men who had a previous heart attack were slightly less likely to have a recurring heart attack. Niacin use is also associated with arrhythmias, suggesting that niacin should not be used if you already have heart disease.

In large scientific studies, only 50 to 60 percent of the subjects were able to tolerate the side effects of the mega doses of this agent needed to reduce lipids. It causes flushing, which may be experienced as hot flashes or severe itching. Also, hepatitis, gout, peptic ulcers, and a reduced ability to control diabetes have been reported. Newer treatments, such as statins, are now the preferred drugs for reducing cholesterol. However, if your cholesterol is still high while taking one of the newer statin drugs, your physician may recommend you add niacin to your regimen.

The most common form of niacin medication is niacin-extended release (Niaspan, Advicor).

Nitrates

Nitrate-containing drugs such as nitroglycerine are the oldest class of drugs used for shortening and preventing painful angina attacks. They come in many formulations: sublingual tablet, patch, ointment, spray, and intravenous solution. They are often used for quick relaxation of constricted blood vessels, such as just before exercising or after a heart attack in an attempt to prevent further damage, or death. They are delivered into the smooth muscle cells of your blood vessels and are then converted into nitrous oxide, a powerful dilator of blood vessels, which causes them to relax.

These nitrates dilate not only the arteries of your body, including the coronary arteries, but also your veins. This causes a redistribution of some of the blood from your heart into your veins so that there is less blood in the heart, thereby presenting your heart with a smaller volume of blood to push out into the arteries, and therefore reducing strain on the heart. The dilation of the arteries also reduces the resistance your heart encounters when it tries to pump blood out into the body. Both of these cause a decrease in the workload of the heart, and reduce its need for oxygen. With dilated blood vessels, blood can also more easily flow through partially blocked coronary arteries to bring a greater supply of oxygen to your heart. All of these contribute to stopping the pain of angina, and reducing your heart's craving for oxygen and important nutrients.

For people who have had a heart attack, nitrates have been used to help them live through the days following a heart attack. Nitrates don't affect the clot that has caused the heart attack, but they can release the tightness of the arteries around the blockage and reduce the effects of the heart attack. Nitrates are usually used for short-term purposes, as their effects wear off quickly.

Examples of the most frequently prescribed nitrate-containing drugs are isosorbide dinitrate (Isordil, Dilatrate-SR), isosorbide mononitrate (Imdur, Imso, Monoket), nitroglycerin sublingual (Nitrostat), nitroglycerin spray (Nitrolingual), nitroglycerin patch (Nitro-Dur, Transdur-Nitro), and nitroglycerin ointment (Nitro-Bid).

Nitrates cause fewer harmful side effects than many of the other drugs used for cardiovascular problems. Yet, like all modern drugs, there are some negative effects associated with their use. One common side effect is headache. Headaches occur when blood vessels in the brain become dilated. People have reported throbbing headaches shortly after the administration of this drug.

Feeling dizzy and lightheaded are two other side effects frequently experienced when taking nitrates. Normally the veins in the legs constrict when you stand up. This stops blood from pooling in your legs. Nitrates reduce this ability of your veins to tighten, which may cause you to feel dizzy or even faint when you get up after lying down or sitting.

Other undesirable effects include rapid pulse, nausea, and reddening and warming of the skin due to a greater amount of blood flowing into the small vessels in your skin. Most people have a problem tolerating nitrates to some degree.

Thrombolytic Drugs

Thrombolytic, or clot-busting, drugs are often used in emergency situations to save the life of an individual who has had a heart attack and to help prolong life afterward. As their name suggests, their value in times of cardiac crises comes from their ability to dissolve clots in blood vessels, the primary cause of most heart attacks and the death that often follows. This class of drugs must be injected directly into the bloodstream.

Thrombolytic drugs dissolve blood clots by attacking fibrin, an elastic protein material in the outer crust that holds the clot together. Once injected into the bloodstream, the drug takes just a few seconds to reach the coronary arteries, where it starts to dissolve the clot. As a result, the blood to the heart cells is able to flow again.

The speed at which this occurs can be critical in reducing the potential damage to the heart muscle. As described earlier, if the life-giving blood supply is cut off from the heart, that area of the heart muscle will die. This happens within six minutes. If the blockage is quickly cleared, it can reduce the amount of damage to the heart. Limiting damage to the heart can reduce serious complications, such as acute heart failure or arrhythmia, events that in and of themselves can cause chronic heart failure and cardiac death.

Some of the more frequently used thrombolytic medications include alteplase (Activase), anistreplase (Eminase), reteplase (Reteplase), streptokinase (Steptase), and tenecteplase (TNKase).

Thrombolytic agents are not lightweight medications. Although they can save your life, they can take it away as well. Their clot-busting ability increases the chances of bleeding in the brain and can lead to a stroke. On average, 1 in 250 people have a stroke from the use of thrombolytic drugs. These drugs may also cause you to bleed more easily from an injury or cut, including during surgery. One in ten people who take thrombolytics have serious problems with bleeding. When this happens, a blood transfusion is usually needed. Thrombolytics are also incompatible with many other drugs, herbs, and some foods.

Aspirin

Aspirin is an over-the-counter drug used by millions of people for relieving fever, inflammation, and pain. In more recent years, it has become a very popular drug for the prevention of heart attacks. Aspirin suppresses production of a powerful enzyme in the body called *thromboxane A2.* Normally, thromboxane A2 causes the sticky platelets in blood to aggregate or form clots when you are injured. It also causes the blood vessels to constrict. Unfortunately, when these platelets form clots in the coronary blood vessels that supply your heart muscle, a heart attack can occur. This is of particular concern in atherosclerotic arteries that have already been narrowed.

By blocking the effect of thromboxane A2, aspirin helps the arteries relax and widen, and clot formation in your blood is discouraged, causing improvement of blood flow. Research has shown that taking aspirin during a heart attack or for at least one month after a heart attack reduces your chance of having another heart attack or stroke by one-third. Research has also shown that taking aspirin while experiencing a heart attack increases your probability of living through it. Physicians usually recommend that aspirin taken for these purposes should be continued for several years or for life to prevent another heart attack or stroke.

Just because aspirin is available without a prescription does not mean that it is harmless, even in low doses. Aspirin can cause serious side effects, such as ulcers and bleeding in the intestines and stomach. When severe, these side effects can be life threatening, and they have been responsible for many people needing hospital care or even dying. Irritation to the lining of the stomach may be experienced as indigestion, which may have serious health consequences if prolonged. However, if taken on a full stomach and in a moderate dose, the possibility of these adverse effects can be greatly reduced for the majority of people.

Hormone Replacement Therapy

Before menopause, women generally have a much lower incidence of heart attacks than men, but they catch up with men after the onset of menopause. Aware of this phenomenon, medical researchers explored hormone therapy as a method for reducing fatal heart disease in postmenopausal women. Hormone replacement therapy (HRT or HT) includes hormones that are significantly decreased after the onset of menopause, notably estrogen and progesterone. It was thought that taking these hormones would not only relieve the discomforts of menopause but would also help to reduce a woman's risk of bone loss, heart attacks, and prevent degradation of mental functioning as she ages.

Studies of women taking hormone treatment have shown that hormone therapy in the form of estrogen alone (for example, Premarin) or combined with progesterone (Prempro, Premphase, Ortho-Prefest) can be effective in lessening hot flashes, vaginal dryness, depression, and other discomforts of menopause, and treatment seems to lower the risk of osteoporosis. Unfortunately, the risks may be far greater than the benefits.

Researchers are now finding that when estrogen replacement is taken, women are more likely to have a heart attack or stroke in the first year or two after starting treatment. However, recent clinical trials suggest that taking estrogen and progesterone combined may turn out to be riskier than taking estrogen alone. Moreover, both approaches are fraught with similar side effects. Not only does hormone therapy cause vaginal discharge, but it can also cause uterine bleeding and breast pain. Of even greater concern is increased risk of breast cancer, blood clots, heart disease, and stroke.

SURGICAL PROCEDURES

When drugs cannot alleviate the effects caused by a narrowing or blockage in the coronary arteries, more aggressive approaches are pursued. These are discussed below.

Angioplasty

Angioplasty, or percutaneous coronary intervention (PCI), is a surgical procedure that is generally performed when a narrowing in the coronary artery causes continuous angina pain that cannot be alleviated by drugs. This pain is a sign that the heart is not getting enough oxygen because sufficient blood is not able to get through the blood vessel to give the heart muscle what it needs. This is usually the result of buildup of atherosclerotic plaque in a coronary artery. Angioplasty is also frequently performed when an angiogram (a procedure that allows doctors to visualize blood flow through the heart's arteries) shows significant narrowing in one coronary vessel.

During an angioplasty procedure, a balloon is inserted into the artery and then inflated to open up the blockage. A thin tube called a *catheter* with a balloon on the tip is inserted into an artery in the groin or arm and then threaded up through the blood vessels of the leg, abdomen, or chest, through the aorta, and then into the coronary artery that is blocked. When the balloon reaches the narrowing, the doctor pumps it up, which crushes the hardened fatty plaque against the inner walls of the artery.

Unfortunately, in 30 to 40 percent of people who undergo this procedure, the opened artery eventually returns to its narrowed state. This is called *restenosis*. A new addition to angioplasty is to place a stent into the artery during the surgery to try to prevent this reoccurrence of narrowing. The stent is a stainless-steel mesh tube placed around the balloon that expands with the balloon, and when thought to be sufficiently expanded for blood to pass through, is left behind, acting like a scaffolding to keep the artery open. The balloon is then deflated and removed from the artery, along with the catheter.

An even more recent technological innovation is to coat the stents with drugs that reduce the growth of new cellular scar tissue around the stent. These drug-releasing stents may reduce restenosis rates to 10 to 20 percent. If you have a stent, your physician will likely give you drugs to stop blood clots from forming around it.

Angioplasty surgery normally takes between sixty and ninety minutes and requires a two- to three-day hospital stay. A series of studies have shown that angioplasty may provide relief from symptoms of angina more effectively than drug therapy in selected patients. However, this procedure has not been shown to prevent heart attacks or death more than nonsurgical medical therapy. Yet, more than 3 million angioplasties are performed in the United States every year at a cost of $10,000 to $15,000 each. It has been suggested by some medical experts that many of these procedures are unnecessary and costly. For individuals with heart disease and with no or mild symptoms of angina, aggressive nonsurgical therapy is often preferable.

Although many people experience relief of their symptoms after angioplasty surgery, there are many complications and risks both during and after surgery that need to be considered. During surgery, the patient may experience chest pain, heavier bleeding with a big bruise afterward, and an infection where the needle was inserted. Also, although rare, the catheter can injure, cut, or puncture the artery, causing the need for immediate surgery to correct the complications. A more common occurrence is bleeding plaque, injury to the cells lining the artery wall, and blood clots as a result of the inside of the artery being touched or scraped by the balloon or stent.

Other serious risks may arise during surgery. These may include allergic reaction to the dyes that are used; the need to keep repeating the procedure several times if there is difficulty getting the artery sufficiently open; a narrowing in the artery that is too long or too tight to be operated on; a sudden closing of the artery that causes a heart attack during or just after the procedure (in 3 to 5 out of 100 cases); emergency open heart surgery to bypass the area if the blockage is bad (2 out of 100); emergency coronary artery bypass grafting if the blockage is made worse by the procedure (5 out of 100); a stroke right after angioplasty (1 out of 100); major bleeding (7 out of 100); and death (1 out of 100). These rates for complications are higher for elderly people, and are even higher if you go to a physician or hospital that does not routinely perform many of these procedures.

One last risk you may want to consider. Remember the influence of injury in the development of atherosclerosis? It is thought that the scraping and injury in the artery due to angioplasty contribute to the development of atherosclerosis in the artery, and may participate in the high rate of restenosis in angioplasty patients.

Coronary Artery Bypass Graft Surgery

Coronary artery bypass graft (CABG) surgery is a more invasive procedure than angioplasty and is also used for overcoming the effects of blockage of the coronary arteries. It is primarily performed in cases where the blockage is so significant or recalcitrant that a detour around it (a bypass) is needed to sufficiently increase the flow of blood around the heart. Your physician may suggest bypass surgery for the following reasons:

- You have chest pain whenever you exert yourself physically.

- You still have chest pain even though you are taking drugs for angina.

- An angiogram shows narrowing of your coronary arteries, particularly if all three of them are narrowed, or if your heart's main artery (left main coronary artery) is involved.

- The left side (left ventricle) of your heart is not working very well.

- The narrow part of your artery cannot be successfully widened by angioplasty.

Coronary artery bypass is accomplished by taking sections of healthy blood vessels from some other part of the body and grafting them onto the narrowed coronary artery, including areas both before and after the area of blockage. The blood vessels used for this surgery are often taken from the leg (the saphenous vein), inside the chest (internal mammary artery), and/or the arm (radial artery). It is very common for people to need more than one graft. In fact, most people need three or four.

Studies that have followed heart patients for several years after angioplasty or bypass surgery show that heart attack and death rates are similar. However, bypass surgery has been shown to be helpful in reducing the incidence of future heart attacks and death in individuals with severe symptoms that are resistant to nonsurgical therapy; in individuals who have major narrowing in their left main coronary artery or in all three main coronary vessels; and in individuals with poor pumping capacity of the heart.

Each year more than 1 million coronary bypass surgeries are performed worldwide—with 500,000 done in the United States alone—at an average cost of $30,000 to $50,000. It has been suggested that, like angioplasties, many of these procedures are performed unnecessarily and that their major side effects and high cost might be avoided with more intensive uses of nonsurgical approaches.

There are many risks and complications that can occur during and right after the surgery, and for some time afterward. During surgery, there are rare and very serious cases of people who are allergic to the anesthetics that are used. One-third of bypass surgery patients usually need blood transfusions to replace lost blood. Five in one hundred of these patients will bleed so profusely that they will require an emergency operation to stop the bleeding. Three in one hundred will have a new heart attack during or just after surgery. In older individuals or in those who have had a prior bypass operation, the mortality rate rises to four to eight people in one hundred.

You could be among the 30 percent of people who, after having this procedure, will develop an arrhythmia and will need to take drugs to stay alive. In addition, you may have a hard time breathing right after surgery and will be among the one in ten who need a ventilator machine to breathe. It has also been found that five in one hundred people may have a stroke or other permanent neurological damage. More than 30 percent of people suffering a stroke after surgery die. Your kidneys may also stop working properly; and although most people recover, there are rare cases in which a dialysis machine is permanently needed to remove waste material from your blood.

Because of the extreme invasiveness of this surgery to the heart, chest, and extremities, if a blood vessel is removed, it takes months for the body to heal. Usually you will need strong pain medication for several weeks afterward. You could also be the one to five out of one hundred who will develop memory or other cognitive problems for six months or longer, or among the one in seven out of one hundred who will have a heart attack within thirty days. Unfortunately, follow-up research has also found that three in one hundred people die within thirty days after receiving bypass surgery.

After all this, three in ten patients will still have angina after the surgery. And within five years, angina will return to five in ten patients.

CONCLUSION

The unfortunate outcome of conventional strategies for heart health is that despite all the drugs and surgery used, the real cause of the disease is never addressed. Conventional strategies are like a bandage put on top of a deep wound, without the process that needs to occur for that wound to heal and bring you back to a state of well-being and health. Underneath all the rerouting of coronary arteries, and the makeshift and damaging approaches of modern drugs and surgery, the silent and deadly advance of your heart disease takes place.

This chapter has touched on the major drugs and surgical procedures that are used by conventional medicine to treat and/or prevent heart disease. What is apparent is that all modern drugs and surgical procedures carry with them risks of harmful side effects and that none of these approaches deal with the ultimate cause of heart disease. In the next section, we will investigate the basis of heart disease more deeply and describe how a series of simple and natural approaches can effectively and safely create total heart health.

II. The Total Heart Health Program

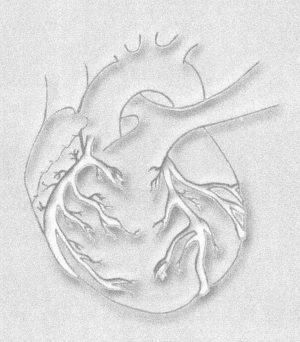

❦ CHAPTER 4 ❦

A New Strategy for Total Heart Health: The Maharishi Vedic Approach to Health

THE MAHARISHI VEDIC APPROACH TO HEALTH is the restoration of the world's most ancient system of natural health care. It is a unique, sophisticated, comprehensive system of scientific knowledge and self-care technologies that considers factors that influence your health at all levels—from your innermost mind, to your physical body, to your immediate surroundings of home and community, to the outermost reaches of the cosmos. It connects all these levels to the intelligence that lies deep within you, at the basis of your mind and body.

Because of this connectivity that promotes heart health at its most basic and holistic level, the Total Heart Health program is uniquely effective and free of harmful side effects. In contrast, modern medicine does not provide this depth and range of benefits, addressing for the most part only the symptoms of chronic diseases using diagnostic and therapeutic modalities that are typically associated with harmful or even lethal side effects.

As discussed in Section I, the ability of modern medicine to treat or prevent heart disease and its risk factors is limited and inadequate. Conventional treatments address symptoms and, on occasion, the biochemistry or anatomy underlying the symptoms, but they do not address the ultimate causes of heart disease and clearly don't eliminate them.

In contrast, the Maharishi Vedic Approach to Health addresses the quantum mechanical imbalances that precede and cause disease and suffering. In the case of heart disease (or any disease for that matter), the development of imbalances and, subsequently, of clinical disorders is due to the body's inability to access its own inner intelligence. Providing this missing link makes the Vedic approach distinctively effective and free from harmful side effects.

As you may remember, in Vedic literature this inner intelligence of the body or *inner self* is a unified field, called *Atma.* Through its own self-interacting dynamics, this deepest level of nature's functioning gives rise to all the diverse laws of physics, chemistry, biology, astronomy, and so on that create and maintain order in the entire universe. All these laws of nature are contained in the verses of the *Veda,* a term that means, in the ancient language of Sanskrit, "complete knowledge." Because all the laws of nature emerge from within the unified field through its own self-interacting dynamics, these laws that govern the entire universe are all unified at their source. Therefore, this unified field of natural law is the intelligence of nature within you and everything in the universe, including your body.

MODERN SCIENCE CORROBORATES ANCIENT VEDIC SCIENCE

Quantum physics, considered to be the most advanced level of modern science, is now confirming the view cognized by the ancient Vedic scientists of the fundamental structure of the universe and its emergence from a unified field. Like these early Vedic scientists, modern physicists define the unified field as a single, universal source of all orderliness in nature.

It is only within the past several decades that quantum physicists have discovered that the structure of the universe and how it operates are fundamentally different from what we previously thought. Today, quantum physicists think that all matter and energy in the universe when reduced to its finest level—the quantum level—is composed of forces and/or energies interconnected by a single unified field of natural law. According to leading quantum physicist Dr. John Hagelin, "It was [originally] Einstein's deep conviction that the laws of nature had a simple, geometric, unified foundation, and that this unification could be understood by the human intellect. Within the past [four] decades, a number of important breakthroughs in this area have led to a progressively more unified understanding of the laws of nature, culminating in the recent discovery of completely unified field theories."

The unified field is an unmanifest, invisible field of energy and intelligence that, through interaction with itself, gives rise to all the laws of nature responsible for the manifestation and administration of the entire universe. It is the nonmaterial basis of all material things. It includes all physical phenomenon from the subatomic level of protons, neutrons, and electrons, which make up atoms and molecules, to the body's cells, tissues and organs, to the cosmic level containing the sun, moon, stars, planets, and galaxies.

Figure 4.1 illustrates the unmanifest unified field of all the laws of nature from which the fundamental force and matter fields emerge to provide the basis for the physical world, including our own physiology. All forms and phenomena in the universe, all the laws of the various sciences, sequentially emerge from this field. It is a level where, as the name implies, these laws of science are unified at their source.

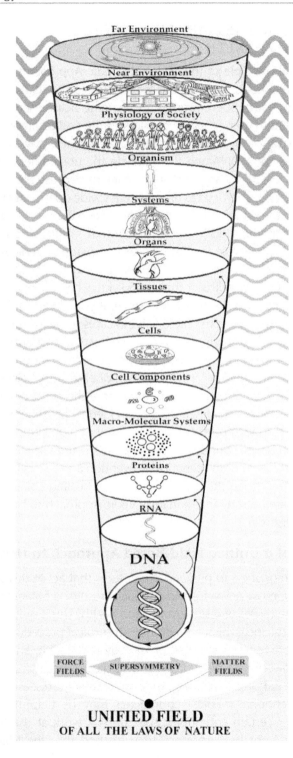

Figure 4.1.
Unified Field
Chart for Total
Heart Health

UNIQUENESS OF THE MAHARISHI VEDIC
APPROACH TO HEALTH

The fundamental principle of the Maharishi Vedic Approach to Health is that the body naturally heals itself once it is reconnected to its own inner intelligence. How does this happen? From this viewpoint, heart disease—or any type of disorder for that matter—may be considered the end result of a loss of functioning in accordance with the basic blueprint of one's physiology, which is found in each person's DNA and ultimately in the unified field at the basis of our physiologies. Heart disease insidiously develops because the body gradually forgets how to keep the structures of the arteries wide open, how to keep blood flowing with just the right pressure, and how to keep the heart beating in a way that maintains a rhythm and pumping ability that satisfies and is coordinated with the needs of the rest of the body. In the language of Vedic science, this is due to the loss of memory of one's own inner intelligence or Atma.

A healthy heart is an indicator that an individual has a strong and lively connection to his or her body's inner intelligence. If you already suffer from heart disease or one or more of its risk factors, it indicates some loss of connection to your natural healing mechanisms. To prevent heart disease from occurring in the first place, the Maharishi Vedic Approach to Health recognizes physiological imbalances before the clinical symptoms of disease arise, before the onset of chest pain or shortness of breath, and long before the onset of a sudden heart attack or stroke. This system of health care can identify physiological imbalances even before the diagnosis of high blood pressure or high cholesterol shows up in an exam or lab test in your doctor's office. Exactly the same model is used to reverse heart disease. In both scenarios, prevention and reversal, the strategy is to restore and strengthen the body's own innate healing abilities. Indeed, the same principles are used by the Maharishi Vedic Approach to Health to address any disease or disorder.

Advantages of a Unified Field-Based Approach to Heart Health

Introducing therapeutic and preventive measures that act at this subtle level of life produces the most powerful and beneficial results: a balanced physiology, elimination of the causes of disease, and good health. This is quite different from conventional medicine, which uses drugs and surgical procedures to intervene at gross and more material levels of physiology and health, and which is considerably less powerful. At best, drugs and surgical procedures only reduce or cover up disease symptoms; at worst, they can cause new disease or even death.

While conventional medical approaches may be helpful for alleviating symptoms under certain conditions, they do not work at the foundation of disease. It should not be surprising, then, to find that the Maharishi Vedic

Approach to Health can treat and even reverse heart disease more effectively than can modern medicine alone. As noted throughout this book, this finding is backed up by hundreds of scientific studies and the clinical experience of several million people around the world.

Nor is it surprising that conventional medicine's view of disease does not consider the body's own inner intelligence, which operates and coordinates the myriad molecules, cells, tissues, organs, and systems in the body. After all, the unified field is the subtlest level of nature. Just as the vastness of the ocean is hidden under the waves at the surface—and one has to dive into it to appreciate its depths—so the silent field of the body's inner intelligence is hidden beneath the endless activity of the human physiology.

Approaching human health without knowledge of this underlying intelligence is like building or repairing a house without referring to the blueprints. The wiring and plumbing could be installed or redone incorrectly. All sorts of errors in the house's structure and function might occur. So it is with your heart's health. When the knowledge of the unified field is missing as a consequence of incomplete knowledge, errors in structure and function in the cardiovascular system and whole body occur, and the result is the onset of disease and suffering. As the errors accumulate, the potential for harm increases.

Focusing on the fundamental basis of heart disease gives the Maharishi Vedic Approach to Health another advantage. It recognizes imbalances that lead to disease at their earliest stages and is therefore able to more effectively reverse those imbalances. Modern medicine, in contrast, usually recognizes diseases only at later stages, after they have become symptomatic, such as when you go to the doctor with a complaint. Even screening for high blood pressure or high cholesterol turns up disorders only after they have already exceeded a threshold level. These disorders are but the tip of the iceberg; the entire iceberg—the disease or disorder—has, by the time it has been discovered by modern medicine, been there a long time, lurking beneath the surface.

Attempts to understand the origin of disease is occurring in some venues of modern medical research. For instance, present-day scientists are attempting to decode the human genome. This is a national effort consuming a great many resources. This search means looking in the DNA molecule for the code behind all physiological processes, and hoping to determine why health is lost and diseases like heart disease occur. While this approach is going in the right direction, that is, searching for ways to prevent and treat heart disease at more subtle and profound levels, it does not go nearly deep enough. Because the traditional Vedic perspective describes the patterns of intelligence at the basis of the human body, patterns that give rise to all specific physiological expressions of the body, it can be said to have already decoded the human genome. In this

TABLE 4.1. FORTY ASPECTS OF VEDA AND VEDIC LITERATURE IN HUMAN PHYSIOLOGY		
BRANCH	EXPRESSION IN THE HUMAN PHYSIOLOGY	
1	Rik Veda	Whole Physiology
2	Sama Veda	Sensory Systems
3	Yajur Veda	Processing Systems
4	Atharva Veda	Motor Systems
5	Shiksha	Autonomic Ganglia
6	Kalpa	Limbic System
7	Vyakarana	Hypothalamus
8	Nirukta	Autonomic Nervous System and Pituitary Gland
9	Chhandas	Neurohormones, Neurotransmitters
10	Jyotish	Basal Ganglia, Deep-seated Nuclei
11	Nyaya	Thalamus
12	Vaisheshika	Cerebellum
13	Samkhya	Cells, Tissues, Organs
14	Yoga	Cerebral Cortex
15	Karma Mimansa	Central Nervous System
16	Vedanta	Integrated Functioning of the Nervous System
17	Gandharva Veda	Cycles and Rhythms
18	Dhanur Veda	Biochemistry, Enzymes, Immune System, Vertebral Column
19	Sthapatya Veda	Anatomy

light, the Maharishi Vedic Approach to Health is the fulfillment of modern molecular medicine. Indeed, the Vedic system may be considered an *ultra modern* system of medicine because it works at the most fundamental level of the physiology—quantum physics—which is also the most advanced level of modern science. It is knowledge of this level that forms the basis of principles and practices that comprise the Total Heart Health program outlined in upcoming chapters.

DISCOVERY OF VEDA AND THE VEDIC LITERATURE IN HUMAN PHYSIOLOGY

In addition to modern science's confirmation of the presence and importance

BRANCH	EXPRESSION IN THE HUMAN PHYSIOLOGY	
20	Harita Samhita	Venous and Biliary Systems
21	Bhela Samhita	Lymphatic System, Glial Cells
22	Kashyapa Samhita	Arterial System
23	Charaka Samhita	Cell Nucleus
24	Sushruta Samhita	Cytoplasm, Cell Organelles
25	Vagbhata Samhita	Cytoskeleton, Cell Membrane
26	Madhava Nidan Samhita	Mesodermal Tissues
27	Shamgadhara Samhita	Endodermal Tissues
28	Bhava Prakasha Samhita	Ectodermal Tissues
29	Upanishad	Ascending Tracts of the Central Nervous System
30	Aranyaka	Fasciculi Proprii
31	Brahamana	Descending Tracts of the Central Nervous System
32	Itihasa	Voluntary Motor and Sensory Projections
33	Purana	Great Intermediate Net
34	Smriti	Memory Systems, Reflexes
35	Rik Veda Pratishakhya	Cerebral Cortex, Layer 1
36	Shukla Yajur Veda Pratishakhya	Cerebral Cortex, Layer 2
37	Atharva Veda Pratishakhya	Cerebral Cortex, Layer 5
38	Atharva Veda Pratishakhya (chaturadhayi)	Cerebral Cortex, Layer 6
39	Krishna Yajur Veda Pratishakya	Cerebral Cortex, Layer 3
40	Sama Veda Pratishakya	Cerebral Cortex, Layer 4

of a unified field of all the laws of nature, another remarkable discovery with far-reaching implications was made during the past ten years, this time by a great neuroscientist, Professor Tony Nader, M.D., Ph.D.

Professor Nader discovered one-to-one correlations between the detailed descriptions of the human body and its many divisions, subdivisions, and processes found in the ancient Vedic literature, and the divisions, subdivisions, and processes discovered by modern scientific research on physiology, from organ systems down to the level of DNA molecules. He found that every division (structure) and every process (function) understood by modern physiology has an exact counterpart within the divisions and descriptions provided by the ancient Vedic literature. Table 4.1 lists the forty traditional branches of the Vedic literature and their correlations with the major branches of human physiology as discovered by Professor Nader.

To help explain this concept, consider the branch of the Vedic literature called *Gandharva Veda* (Branch 17 in Table 4.1). Gandharva Veda represents harmony in nature. On one level, Gandharva Veda can be thought of as music, whether voice or instrumental. One may listen to a *raga*, or musical piece, that is specifically suited to the time of day or purpose of the event, such as celebration or relaxation. On another level, Gandharva Veda music is expressed in the human physiology as the cycles and rhythms that keep the body in tune with the rhythms of nature. These rhythms include the secretion of hormones, metabolism, the rhythm of the heart and circadian rhythms of blood pressure, heart rate, and other well-organized patterns in cardiovascular physiology. Because of the one-to-one correspondence noted above, listening to Gandharva Veda music helps reconnect the body's physiology to the cycles and rhythms of its own inner intelligence. This restores balance and resets the system.

Professor Nader's discovery validated the ancient Vedic concept of total health in a way that is consistent with modern science, yet it extends beyond the limited boundaries of modern medicine's understanding of the body and of health. It shows that the laws that give structure to the many facets of the Veda and Vedic literature are the same laws of nature that express themselves in the human body and, indeed, throughout the whole universe.

The practical significance of Professor Nader's discovery is enormous. It means that the field of Veda, the unified field of natural law that structures and governs the whole universe, is deep within you as a blueprint for the orderly functioning and perfect health of your body. Furthermore, this intelligence within you, which is the intelligence of nature, is not only fundamental to your body, but it is also fundamental to everything else that influences your health, including your mind and your environment. What is needed is to apply those approaches from within each of these areas of life that most effectively allow your inner intelligence to be fully expressed in your physiology.

The Maharishi Vedic Approach to Health provides forty approaches that arise from each of the forty different aspects of the Veda and Vedic literature. Each area of knowledge has associated technologies of the unified field. With these technologies or practical methods, not only can you attend to each of the different areas of the body that are associated with the particular aspect of the Vedic literature, but also each approach helps you to restore areas in your mind, body, or environment that may not be in harmony with your inner intelligence, the unified field of natural law.

As we discussed above, each of us carries within ourselves a copy of this blueprint of natural law—a precise set of plans that will allow us to achieve total health. Professor Nader's discovery shows how, through approaches associated with each of the forty different aspects of the Vedic literature, you can tend to every aspect of your health. The Total Heart Health program provides the practical techniques and practices for heart disease prevention and reversal that are associated with this knowledge. Each approach helps establish a reference point for health in the unified field located deep within your physiology. As you begin to tap your own inner intelligence, your innate potential will become more available to you, and imbalances—even long-standing ones—will be eliminated and your heart and body will begin to heal. Over time, the end result will be that optimal health becomes your everyday reality.

GETTING STARTED

The remainder of the book is dedicated to presenting the diagnostic and therapeutic modalities of the Total Heart Health program. The modalities can be categorized into three broad approaches: the Mind Approach, the Body Approach, and the Environment Approach. The following are brief descriptions of each section. Remember that each approach by itself has been shown to be effective for preventing and treating heart disease. Therefore, you may take advantage of one or all of them according to your circumstances. Research has shown that using a comprehensive multi-modality Total Heart Health program results in benefits that are greater than a single modality. The choice is always yours to begin from where you are.

The Mind Approach

A cornerstone of the Total Heart Health program is the Transcendental Meditation program. It is the most powerful means for reducing stress, enhancing mind-body coordination, and restoring the inner intelligence of the unified field to the functioning of your mind and body. Hundreds of scientific studies have shown that the Transcendental Meditation technique reduces psychological stress and its physiological consequences and helps create better mental, emotional, physical, and social health. This simple, natural program is a powerful means for bringing balance to your entire physiology for total health.

The Body Approach

The Body Approach for heart disease and its major risk factors includes recommendations for diet, herbal food supplements, exercise, daily and seasonal routines, and physiological purification therapies all designed to remove the obstacles to the flow of your own inner intelligence. Each of these recommendations takes the approach of enlivening the unified field that is at the basis of your physiology and, in the process, restores the orderly and balanced functioning of your mind and body.

The Environment Approach

The environment has a dramatic and profound effect on both physical and mental health. Environmental pollutants have been shown to cause cardiovascular disease and mortality. Crime, violence, and war also affect the mind, body, and heart. The Environment Approach addresses these influences on health and offers practical ways to balance both your near and distant environment. These include Vedic sound therapies to align the body's rhythms with nature's rhythms; Vedic architecture for healthy, life-supporting homes and offices; consideration of the stress levels in your community; and knowledge and technologies to diagnose and utilize the cycles and rhythms of nature for total heart health.

PART ONE

The
Mind
Approach

❦ CHAPTER 5 ❦

Healing Your Heart
Through the Mind

OVER THE PAST FORTY YEARS, SCIENTIFIC RESEARCH has repeatedly demonstrated that your mind affects your body and health. In the Total Heart Health program, the Transcendental Meditation program is considered the single most important modality in the Mind Approach for improving overall health. It is a simple, natural technique that restores access to the body's own inner intelligence. With regular practice, this technique leads to integration and balance of mind and body. Hundreds of studies worldwide on the Transcendental Meditation program consistently confirm its wide range of stress-reducing and health-promoting effects, including its ability to reduce the risk factors for heart disease, prevent and treat the life-threatening effects of this disease, and be instrumental in reversing it.

Accoording to traditional Vedic science, the unified field, through its own self-interacting dynamics, structures all physical and nonphysical phenomena in the universe. From this perspective, the most basic level of the mind is also the unified field. The human mind is described by Vedic scientists as arising from the unified field in the same way that the elementary particles form from the fundamental quantum fields of energy and matter. As Robert Keith Wallace, Ph.D., describes in his book *The Physiology of Consciousness*, the subjective mental structures of consciousness (that is, the mind) may also be regarded as the major modes of expression of the underlying field of pure consciousness, or the unified field. The mind and body have the same source, one unified field of natural law. Therefore, "subjectivity and objectivity are not separate, discrete aspects of life, never to be reconciled; they are merely different themes of the same fundamental field of life."

Furthermore, according to Maharishi Mahesh Yogi as described in his book *The Science of Being and Art of Living,* the mind lies between the unified field and the body. That is, it may be said that the mind is a nonphysical expression of the unified field, which then becomes more manifested or crystallized in physical forms of matter and energy, which in turn make up the physiology of our body. Thus, from this perspective, the state of the mind has a great influence on the state of the body and health.

THE MIND'S ROLE IN HEART DISEASE

As mentioned in Chapter 2, chronic exposure to stressful situations is associated with increased rates of hypertension and heart disease. Job strain, family stress, major losses, other life changes, social isolation, and any situation in which we perceive a threat to our well-being are all major stressors. Our chronic responses to these stressful situations, which may manifest as anxiety, anger, fear, or depression, also add to this increased risk for cardiovascular disease.

One way stress is translated into disorders in your cardiovascular system is through the body's stress-response systems. These systems can become overactive during chronically stressful situations. One of these systems is called the *hypothalamic-pituitary-adrenal axis,* or HPA axis, an important part of the body's neurohormonal system. In stressful situations, the hypothalamus in the brain signals the pituitary gland to release factors that cause the adrenal glands to increase their release of the powerful stress hormone cortisol. The other system is called the *sympathetic nervous system* or the *"fight-or-flight" response.* In stressful situations, an increase in brain activity increases activity in the sympathetic nervous system, which causes the release of the hormones and neurotransmitters epinephrine and norepinephrine, also called *adrenaline* and *noradrenaline.* These excite the heart and cardiovascular system. For example, the heart and blood vessels are stimulated to support the quick fight-or-flight action that is necessary to avoid or address the perceived threat.

If stressful situations are frequently experienced, or are extreme or long lasting, and if our revved-up responses become chronic, that is, if these stress-response systems stay overactive all or most of the time, damage to our tissues and organs can ensue. In particular, this chronic overactivation can stimulate the heart to work harder and the blood vessels to narrow and eventually thicken with plaque. The disruption of the cardiovascular system and other related systems, such as the immune system, leads to heart disease, including hypertension, heart attack, and stroke.

In his book *The End of Stress as We Know It,* neuroscientist Bruce McEwen, Ph.D., describes the effects of prolonged or recurrent stress on the healthy functioning of the brain and body. He introduces the concept of *allostatic load,* which refers to the burden on the nervous system that results from the cumulative effect of chronic stress on the body. As this burden—the allostatic load—increases, it limits your ability to reestablish homeostasis or physiological balance during and after stressful situations. In other words, chronic stress limits your ability to adapt to your environment and makes the body susceptible to heart disease.

Like McEwen and other modern medical scientists, the Maharishi Vedic Approach to Health recognizes the detrimental impacts of stress on the mind and body, but unlike them, it perceives the ultimate cause of the problem differently. According to the Vedic approach, the chronic effects of stress are a sign of blockage in the flow of the body's inner intelligence from its source in the unified field to all parts of your physiology. If expression of the body's own inner know-how can be restored, then stress will have no impact on the body and on the ideal functioning of the heart.

HEALTH BENEFITS OF TRANSCENDENTAL MEDITATION

The Transcendental Meditation program is the most important modality of the Mind Approach used in the Total Heart Health program. When practiced for fifteen to twenty minutes twice a day, this simple, natural, and effortless technique allows the mind to gain deep rest while remaining wide awake. Because of the body's intimate relationship with the mind, the body experiences a corresponding state of deep rest and relaxation. This deep rest increases access to one's inner intelligence, neutralizes existing tensions or stress in both the mind and body, and causes them to become revitalized and enlivened with energy, vitality, intelligence, and creativity.

A vast body of scientific research on the effects of the Transcendental Meditation program conducted by our research institute and at more than 200 universities and research institutes in thirty countries demonstrates that by attending to the mind with this specific technique, you can heal the body as well. The reduction of stress and its physiological consequences manifests in reductions in major risk factors for heart disease, or in the disease itself, and even in longer life span. Following are some of the research findings from our institute and others that demonstrate the positive effects of the Transcendental Meditation program on heart health.

Lowered Stress Hormones

Scientific evidence indicates that the Transcendental Meditation technique works by restoring normal and more ideal functioning in the nervous system, including its two major stress responses systems—the sympathetic nervous system or the fight-or-flight response system, and the neurohormonal system, or the HPA axis. These brain-body systems have major influences on the heart and cardiovascular system. The Transcendental Meditation technique has also been shown to enhance the overall healing ability of the body. This protects the body from the assault of stressful situations and removes and prevents imbalances in the cardiovascular system.

In a study published in the journal *Hormones and Behavior,* Ron Jevning, Ph.D., and colleagues at the University of California–Irvine measured cortisol levels of people while they practiced the Transcendental Meditation technique and compared them with the cortisol levels of a control group. As mentioned, levels of the stress hormone cortisol normally increase during stressful situations. While this increase may be helpful in responding to a physical stress in the short term, chronically elevated cortisol levels end up damaging the blood vessel walls and raising lipid levels. This is one physiological reason why chronically stressed people have more heart disease.

When Dr. Jevning and colleagues compared cortisol levels of subjects practicing the Transcendental Meditation technique (the "meditators") with cortisol levels of subjects in a control group who simply rested with their eyes closed, they found that the average level of cortisol decreased about 33 percent in the meditators during their practice of the technique. The levels of cortisol did not change significantly in the control subjects. (See Figure 5.1.) Indeed, other studies have shown that blood cortisol levels are lowered long term in individuals practicing the Transcendental Meditation program compared to control subjects not practicing the technique.

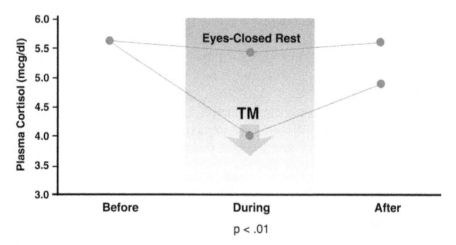

Figure 5.1. Reduced Cortisol During Practice of Transcendental Meditation Technique

Source: Data from *Hormones and Behavior* 10 (1978): 54–60, and *Neuroscience and Biobehavioral Reviews* 16 (1992): 415–424.

Subsequent studies have shown that the ability to maintain lower levels of cortisol and other stress-related hormones such as adrenaline is associated with the length of time, that is, number of months or years, a person has been practicing the Transcendental Meditation program. This indicates that the body can build up resiliency to stressful situations. According to one follow-up study published in the journal *Psychoneuroendocrinology,* researchers at the Institute for Natural Medicine and Prevention observed that after four months of Transcendental Meditation practice, young adults exhibited improved adaptation to stress. These people showed reduced blood cortisol levels in nonstressful situations and enhanced cortisol responses during challenging situations with a rapid return to equilibrium. These findings suggest that the practice of the Transcendental Meditation technique increases a person's ability to adapt to stressful situations through a quicker rise in cortisol and a more rapid recovery after the stressful event has passed.

Other published studies have demonstrated reduced activation of the sympathetic nervous system. This was observed as reductions in levels of adrenaline and noradrenaline circulating in the blood of long-term Transcendental Meditation practitioners. Further research has shown that Transcendental Meditation practitioners have fewer receptors in their body for adrenaline. Receptors act like tiny locks on the surface of cells that receive the key (in this case, adrenaline) and are switched on by it. The fewer number of receptors is beneficial because it leads to less excitation of the sympathetic nervous system. A less excited, more calm and restful nervous system, in turn, will create less damaging effects on the heart and blood vessels.

Research in mind-body medicine has shown that any type of stress, whether it is mental, physical, social, or environmental can have deleterious effects on the heart and the blood vessels through the neurohormonal and sympathetic nervous systems.

Reduced Hypertension

In the late 1980s, a unique collaboration of medical doctors, physiologists, and psychologists at the Institute for Natural Medicine and Prevention and the West Oakland Health Center in Oakland, California, began studying the long-term effects of the Transcendental Meditation program on hypertension and heart disease. The goal was to expand on a series of studies that had been pioneered nearly two decades earlier by neurophysiologist Robert Keith Wallace, Ph.D., at the University of California in Los Angeles, on the physiological effects of the Transcendental Meditation program. Dr. Wallace had found that compared to nonmeditating controls, Transcendental Meditation practitioners had lower metabolic activity, lower blood pressure, and other physiological signs of better health. At the time, few medical scientists had conducted scientifically rigorous controlled studies on the effects of stress reduction on blood pressure.

Over a period of twenty years, we have conducted a series of rigorous clinical studies on the effects of the Transcendental Meditation program on men and women who were at high risk for developing cardiovascular disease or for its recurrence. This research was funded by a series of grants totaling about $20 million from the National Institutes of Health (NIH) and the Retirement Research Foundation (one of the nation's largest foundation for aging research), and other private foundations.

The first study involved 111 people aged fifty-five years and older with mild hypertension, that is, in people with blood pressure over 140/90 mm Hg and less than 160/100 mm Hg on average. Participants were randomly selected to learn either the Transcendental Meditation program or a widely practiced relaxation technique called *progressive muscle relaxation,* or to join a health education control group. Both the Transcendental Meditation and progressive muscle relaxation groups practiced their respective techniques for approximately twenty minutes twice daily. The control group received health-education sessions monthly. Each participant was studied for three months. Blood pressure readings were monitored before, during, and at the end of the study.

The study findings were so amazing that the American Heart Association published the results in their journal *Hypertension* and the popular media carried the story worldwide. The major finding was that the Transcendental Meditation program reduced blood pressure in individuals with mild hypertension at least as effectively as antihypertensive drugs. Among the meditators, the average reduction in blood pressure was 11 mm Hg systolic and 6 mm Hg diastolic. Participants suffered no harmful side effects. Indeed, there were reports of side benefits such as improved psychological health. In addition, the Transcendental Meditation program proved to be twice as effective in lowering blood pressure as progressive muscle relaxation. Blood pressure values in the health-education control group did not change at all (see Figure 5.2).

A follow-up study, published in the *American Journal of Hypertension,* was recently completed by our team at the Institute for Natural Medicine and Prevention on the effects of the Transcendental Meditation program compared with progressive muscle relaxation and conventional health education in people with high blood pressure. This project monitored people with hypertension for a one-year period and showed that those participants who practiced Transcendental Meditation were able to maintain lower blood pressures over the long term. As a result, the meditators were able to reduce their blood pressure medications by about 23 percent compared with the control subjects. This is particularly important because antihypertensive drugs often have unpleasant or

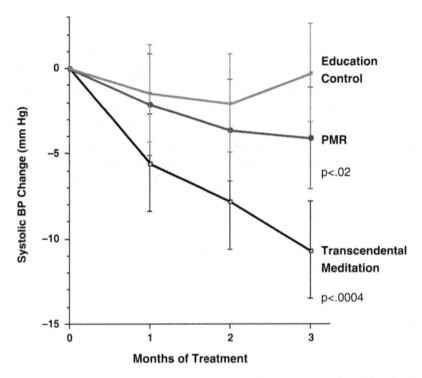

Figure 5.2. Reduction of High Blood Pressure Through the Transcendental Meditation Program

Source: Data from *Hypertension* 26 (1995): 820–827

harmful side effects. The Transcendental Meditation program was found to be highly effective in lowering blood pressure among all major subgroups. It didn't matter whether or not a person's hypertension was associated with obesity, physical inactivity, a high-salt diet, or chronic psychological stress. Other studies have shown that the Transcendental Meditation program lowers high blood pressure in people of widely varying racial and ethnic backgrounds. As Transcendental Meditation instructors are fond of saying, "Anyone who can think a thought can practice the Transcendental Meditation technique and experience beneficial results." The following profile of one of the patients in the early clinical studies is a good example.

As an associate pastor of a Los Angeles church, Betty's daily routine included everything from presiding over church services and functions to overseeing daycare. She also tried to balance her professional life with raising her children and helping in her husband's business. When she was diagnosed with high blood pressure, she decided to do something other than depend on the medications her doctor prescribed.

"It's hard to help others feel good when you don't feel your best yourself," she said. "I couldn't just sit back and be sick."

Betty's doctor recommended that she take part in a unique National Institutes of Health-sponsored study on the effects of the Transcendental Meditation program on hypertension and heart disease. She did some research of her own and found that the Transcendental Meditation program does not involve any lifestyle change, nor did it conflict with her beliefs in any way, and it was the most well-researched stress-management technique around. She signed on immediately as a study participant. She learned the Transcendental Meditation technique, and within one week of regular practice, her blood pressure was normal. Within one month, her doctor cut back her medication.

"I'm back to feeling good about myself and others," she said. "That's the way life is supposed to be lived."

Betty's successful outcome like many others in the studies mentioned above have been replicated by Vernon Barnes, Ph.D., and colleagues at the Medical College of Georgia in Augusta. Only in these studies, the Transcendental Meditation program lowered blood pressure in adolescents with high blood pressure. This finding is particularly important because, in many cases, high blood pressure, like atherosclerosis, begins in childhood or early adulthood. Prevention at this stage can have lifelong benefits.

Lowered Cholesterol and Oxidized Lipids

Several studies have found that cholesterol levels significantly decline with the regular practice of the Transcendental Meditation technique. Remarkably, these changes in cholesterol were not due to alterations in diet because the participants did not change their diets during this study period. So, how can this be explained? Since psychological stress is known to raise cholesterol through the stress hormones cortisol and noradrenaline, it is thought that the practice of the Transcendental Meditation technique may have reduced total cholesterol through its ability to reduce levels of these hormones.

Evidence from studies at the Institute for Natural Medicine and Prevention suggest that the Transcendental Meditation program can reduce the form of cholesterol and other fats in the blood believed to be most responsible for atherosclerosis, that is, oxidized lipids, also called *lipid peroxides.* The research, which was published in *Psychosomatic Medicine,* found that elderly people who practiced the Transcendental Meditation program showed significantly lower levels of lipid peroxides than those who did not, and these differences could not be explained by diet. With lower levels of lipid peroxides in the bloodstream, there is less damage to the artery walls and less buildup of atherosclerotic plaque. There is lower free-radical activity in the body and less artery-clogging material in the blood vessels.

Reduced Psychological Stress

As explained earlier, many types of psychological stress, such as anxiety, depression, anger, and job strain are considered risk factors for hypertension and heart disease. Volumes of research on the Transcendental Meditation program have reported scientific studies on these types of factors. Kenneth Eppley, Ph.D., and colleagues at Stanford University in Palo Alto, California, analyzed the results of 146 studies on the effects of various mind-body techniques on anxiety, the most commonly studied form of psychological stress. These techniques included biofeedback, concentration-type meditation techniques, relaxation techniques such as progressive muscle relaxation, and the Transcendental Meditation technique. The results of this analysis published in the *Journal of Clinical Psychology* showed that the Transcendental Meditation technique was approximately twice as effective in reducing anxiety as other mind-body techniques. The authors of the study suggested that the reason why the Transcendental Meditation program was so effective is because it produces a unique physiological state of restful alertness. This simple yet profound technique restores the mind-body connection, enlivens the body's own inner intelligence, and reduces and eliminates stress (see Figure 5.3).

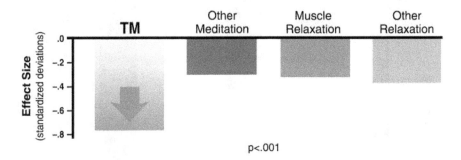

Figure 5.3. Comparison of the Transcendental Meditation Program and Other Mind-Body Techniques for Reducing Stress

Source: Data from *Journal of Clinical Psychology* 45 (1989): 957–974.

Decreased Smoking and Alcohol Abuse

Statistics from the Centers for Disease Control and Prevention indicate that the most preventable cause of death in the United States is cigarette smoking. Smoking is a major risk factor for heart disease because it damages the inside of the blood vessels. Alcohol abuse is another risk factor for heart disease because it damages the heart muscle and raises blood pressure, thereby predisposing heavy drinkers to heart failure, hypertension, arrhythmia, and cardiac mortality.

The Transcendental Meditation program has been shown to naturally prevent and reduce smoking, alcohol, and drug abuse. An analysis of 198 studies by Harvard-trained psychologist Charles Alexander, Ph.D., and colleagues, published in *Alcoholism Treatment Quarterly,* analyzed the effects of different meditation procedures (including the Transcendental Meditation program) and self-development techniques on reducing alcohol, tobacco, and drug abuse. The study reported that the Transcendental Meditation program was three to four times more effective in reducing these forms of substance abuse and thus was by far the most effective. (See Figure 5.4. *Note: "Standard Prevention" refers to conventional education programs and "Standard Treatment" refers to conventional medical programs, such as those that employ nicotine replacement for smoking cessation.)*

The exact physiological mechanisms underlying the ability of the Tran-

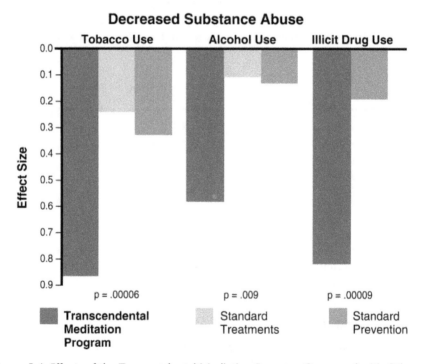

Figure 5.4. Effects of the Transcendental Mediation Program Compared with Other Preventive and Treatment Programs on Smoking, Alcohol, and Drug Abuse

Source: Data from *Alcoholism Treatment Quarterly* 11(1994):13-87.

scendental Meditation technique to achieve such a surprisingly large effect on drug abuse are not known, although reducing stress and creating a more orderly style of functioning in the nervous system are likely to be major factors. Nevertheless, it appears that the Transcendental Meditation program offers a uniquely effective technique for treatment and prevention of smoking, alcohol, and drug abuse, all of which are risk factors for heart disease.

Regression of Atherosclerosis

In the spring 2000 issue of the prestigious medical journal *Stroke,* the American Heart Association published the results of another breakthrough study. This study funded by the NIH and led by Amparo Castillo-Richmond, M.D., at the Institute for Natural Medicine and Prevention. The results were also featured in news reports worldwide. What was so astounding to attract all this attention? This study found that a mind-body technique alone could reduce atherosclerosis and its risk of stroke and heart attack!

In this clinical trial, researchers once again studied African Americans with hypertension. Using ultrasound methods, they measured the thickness of the walls in participants' carotid arteries. The carotid arteries travel up the sides of the neck and carry oxygen to the brain. The thicker the walls of these arteries become, the narrower the opening is for blood to flow through. The same disease process of atherosclerosis that occurs in the coronary arteries leading to the heart and in the arteries leading to the brain, if left unchecked, increases the risk of heart attacks and strokes, respectively.

Participants in the study were divided into two groups. The first group learned the Transcendental Meditation program and practiced for approximately twenty minutes twice daily. The second group attended regular health-education classes for the same period of time. Approximately eight months later, the thickness of the artery walls were measured again in all the participants. Incredibly, in the Transcendental Meditation group, the artery walls had become significantly less thick compared with the health-education group who had *increased* thickening in the artery walls. In other words, the opening inside the arteries, also called the *lumen,* in people practicing the Transcendental Meditation technique had become wider and could carry more blood to the brain—their atherosclerosis had been reversed. The reductions in the thickness of the artery walls induced by Transcendental Meditation practice alone were comparable to reductions achieved by several conventional medications or by intensive diet and exercise programs; yet there were no other lifestyle changes in the Transcendental Meditation group.

Based on studies done by other scientists, this decrease over the first year alone corresponds to an 11 percent reduction in the risk of heart attack and a

15 percent reduction in the risk of stroke in the Transcendental Meditation group compared with control subjects. Presumably additional decreases would be found if the participants were followed over several years. These conclusions were supported by results from a study conducted by John Zamarra, M.D., at the State University of New York–Buffalo and scientists at our institute, and were subsequently published in the *American Journal of Cardiology*. This study found that heart disease patients who would otherwise have been candidates for bypass surgery or angioplasty but chose instead to try the Transcendental Meditation program for about a year showed significant improvements in blood flow to their hearts (a reversal of their myocardial ischemia) and in cardiac function as measured by standard exercise-tolerance testing.

Improved Overall Health

Researcher David Orme-Johnson, Ph.D., of Maharishi University of Management, studied health insurance statistics in over 2,000 people practicing the Transcendental Meditation program over a five-year period. He discovered that Transcendental Meditation practitioners consistently had less than half the number of hospitalizations and doctor visits than did other groups with comparable age, gender, profession, and insurance terms. The difference between the meditation and control groups was even larger among older-age brackets (see Figure 5.5). In addition, people who practiced the Transcendental Meditation technique had lower rates of major diseases in seventeen treatment categories, including 87 percent fewer hospitalizations for heart disease and 55 percent less for cancer. This study demonstrates that practice of the Transcendental Meditation program has a wide range of health-conferring benefits, including prevention of heart disease and other chronic disorders. This is presumably due to the enlivenment of the body's own inner intelligence, resulting in a broad and integrated enhancement of health.

Finally, in a striking follow-up study supported by a grant from the NIH's National Center for Complementary and Alternative Medicine and published in the *American Journal of Cardiology* in 2005, it was demonstrated that people with hypertension from two of our earlier studies, who practiced the Transcendental Meditation program, lived longer compared to other groups with high blood pressure.

An average of eight years after the studies, researchers determined who among the original study participants had died and of what causes. The Transcendental Meditation group showed a 23 percent lower risk of dying overall and a 30 percent lower risk of dying from cardiovascular disease specifically compared with the control groups. This finding on mortality has never been shown for any other mind-body intervention. (See Figure 5.6.)

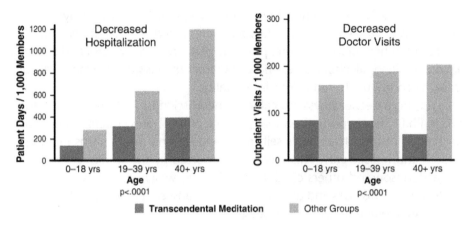

Figure 5.5. Reduced Need for Medical Care by People Practicing the Transcendental
    Meditation Technique

Source: Data from *Psychosomatic Medicine* 49 (1987): 493–507.

There are many possible explanations for the dramatic increase in longevity of the Transcendental Meditation practitioners. Keep in mind that these results are from two randomized-controlled experiments, so it is unlikely that the individuals in the various treatment groups differed from one another enough to account for these major differences in mortality. It was the Transcendental Meditation program that did it. But how exactly?

We believe that there are two ways to explain the physiological and health

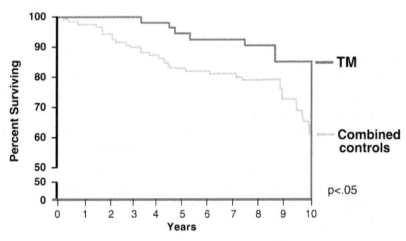

Figure 5.6. Reduced Mortality Rates in Older Men and Women Practicing the
    Transcendental Meditation Program Compared with Controls

Source: Data from the *American Journal of Cardiology* 2005; 95:1060–1064.

effects of the Transcendental Meditation program. First, it is likely that the reductions in cardiovascular risk factors documented in other studies, such as decreases in high blood pressure, psychological stress, cholesterol and oxidized lipids, smoking, alcohol abuse, and even direct markers of coronary heart disease, all contribute to reductions in mortality.

Yet, on a deeper physiological level, neuroscientist Professor Tony Nader, M.D., Ph.D., has hypothesized that practice of the Transcendental Meditation technique restores the body's self-repair and healing mechanisms in an integrated and holistic way. This theory is supported by the studies of Dr. David Orme-Johnson and others cited in this chapter, which show lower rates of a wide range of diseases and disorders among Transcendental Meditation practitioners in addition to less heart disease.

It was further suggested that the profound changes in physiology caused by regular Transcendental Meditation practice were opposite to declines normally found with aging. This idea is consistent with findings of a landmark study published in the mid-1980s by Robert Keith Wallace, Ph.D., who discovered that Transcendental Meditation practice was associated with slowing of physiological aging. Later on, Charles Alexander, Ph.D., then at Harvard University and subsequently co-director of the Institute for Natural Medicine and Prevention, found that older people (average age eighty-one years old) who began the Transcendental Meditation program showed reversals in measures of psychological and physiological aging.

All of these results taken together suggest a holistic effect of the Transcendental Meditation technique that could explain the enhanced longevity that was documented in our study of mortality rates among older Transcendental Meditation practitioners.

CONCLUSION

It is apparent from the more than 600 scientific studies on the health benefits of the Transcendental Meditation technique that the Mind Approach of the Total Heart Health program restores the mind and body's own healing mechanisms to prevent heart disease. These studies show that practicing the Transcendental Meditation technique can help overcome stress-related addictions such as cigarette smoking, and can decrease blood pressure, damaging forms of cholesterol, and atherosclerosis—all of which result in lower rates of disease and a longer life. Examined as a whole, this scientific evidence is proof that practicing Transcendental Meditation is one of the most effective things you can do to achieve total heart health.

In the next chapter, we'll describe in more detail how and why the Transcendental Meditation technique works so well.

CHAPTER 6

How the Transcendental Meditation Program Works

IN THE PREVIOUS CHAPTER, WE SAW THAT EXTENSIVE RESEARCH has verified the health benefits of learning and practicing the Transcendental Meditation technique, the cornerstone of the Mind Approach of the Total Heart Health program. The practice of this technique allows the mind to transcend the thinking process and to experience a unique state of deep rest in body and mind. Simultaneously, a high degree of orderliness or coherence in the brain is gained. Scientists have identified this experience as a fourth major state of consciousness (the first three being sleeping, dreaming, and waking). It is called transcendental consciousness. *It is a natural state that enlivens the body's own inner intelligence. Anyone can learn the practice easily. Courses taught by extensively trained and certified teachers are available in every major city.*

Back when Betty was looking for a natural way to lower her blood pressure, she looked into other stress-reduction techniques for easing the stress in her life, but she discovered that the Transcendental Meditation program was the most efficient means for eliminating stress. (See Betty's story on page 77 in Chapter 5.) Betty knew she could expect to get good results from the program and that it was a truly unique approach and had the best track record available. She found that the outstanding results, as well as the distinctiveness of the Transcendental Meditation technique, had been scientifically verified.

For your own safety and peace of mind, you want to be sure that the health program you choose lives up to its claims of being effective in getting the results you desire. When evaluating any health program, ask these vital questions: Is there scientific evidence for the claims the program makes? What is the program's track record? Has it withstood the test of time by other people? Like Betty, you should find that the Transcendental Medication program has lived up to its claims.

UNIQUENESS OF THE TRANSCENDENTAL MEDITATION TECHNIQUE

Scientific confirmation of the unparalleled effects of the Transcendental Meditation program for enhancing mind-body health was published in the *American Journal of Health Promotion* in 1998. Publication of this article by Drs. David Orme-Johnson and Kenneth G. Walton was particularly exciting because the scope of the study was huge—a review of 600 studies involving more than 20,000 people. The researchers had used meta-analysis and systematic review, rigorous procedures that allow comparison of a wide variety of research designs and measurement scales by creating a standardized measure that can be applied to all studies. "It's like creating a 'common denominator' for the research results from many different universities and research institutions," explains Dr. Orme-Johnson. "Then all the research on different techniques can be directly compared and grand conclusions can be drawn."

What does this particular review of the published scientific research on stress reduction and meditation reveal that has such practical importance for your heart health? It showed that the practice of the Transcendental Meditation program results in greater physiological and psychological health benefits than other forms of meditation and relaxation that have been scientifically studied. This includes progressive relaxation, mindfulness meditation, meditation learned from a book or magazine, biofeedback, traditional practices such as Zen meditation, and self-taught meditation or self-hypnosis. Some examples of the Transcendental Meditation program's distinct effectiveness were discussed in Chapter 5. This objective review of all the published research literature available at the time showed that the Transcendental Meditation program was approximately twice as effective as other modern or traditional relaxation and stress-reduction techniques for reducing blood pressure and anxiety, increasing physiological relaxation and self-actualization, improving psychological outcomes, and decreasing the use of cigarettes, alcohol, and drugs.

In addition, the conclusion reached by Drs. Orme-Johnson and Walton was that the Transcendental Meditation technique, with its basis in the ancient Vedic tradition, is "far more effective than the clinically derived approaches that are modeled after it in reducing anxiety, and improving psychosocial health." It is unparalleled in the benefits it can offer to the mind and body.

When you practice the Transcendental Meditation technique, you naturally begin to experience more settled, or less excited, levels of your own thinking mind, until finally you transcend to the finest, most quiet level of awareness, and experience the unified field of natural law as your own innermost consciousness. At this point, you are experiencing a state of silent wakefulness. In the ancient Vedic tradition, this experience is called *transcendental consciousness.*

EXPERIENCING TRANSCENDENTAL CONSCIOUSNESS

Transcendental consciousness is considered a fourth major state of consciousness, in addition to the three usual states of consciousness you experience daily: waking, dreaming, and sleeping. In this state of transcendental consciousness, you directly experience the unified field at the deepest level of your mind. It is simultaneously the deepest level of your body. As we discussed earlier, this state of transcendental consciousness is considered to be the common ground state of both mind and body, which is why enlivening it through Transcendental Meditation practice has such powerful effects on both mental and physical health. (See Figure 6.1.)

Contrary to popular perception, transcendental consciousness is not a vague or nebulous state. It has been empirically measured and verified by physiological studies in highly sophisticated laboratories. When someone experiences transcendental consciousness, brainwave recordings called electroencephalographs (EEGs) show that the nervous system is deeply relaxed and yet the practitioner is highly alert, in a highly integrated state, as evidenced by measurements of orderliness of brainwave activity, which neuroscientists call coherence. The greater the coherence in the EEG (that is, the greater the synchronization), the more the different parts of the brain are working together. This greater coherence becomes a new style of brain functioning that carries over, after meditating, into daily activities. This is paralleled by increased coherence and orderliness in an individual's behavior as he or she continues to regularly practice the Transcendental Meditation technique over time.

Scientists have shown that the increased orderliness of brain functioning is associated with greater intelligence, creativity, problem-solving ability, and integration of the nervous system. It is also associated with feelings of rest, relaxation, calmness, and peace. Neuroscientists such as Professor Tony Nader, M.D., Ph.D., refer to the experience of transcendental consciousness as "the development of total brain functioning."

Figure 6.2 illustrates early research on the increased coherence in brainwave patterns typically found when people practice the Transcendental Meditation technique daily for shorter (two weeks, left panel) or longer (two years, right panel) periods of time. The figure illustrates that EEG coherence begins within two weeks of practicing the Transcendental Meditation program and increases in amount both during and after meditation over time.

Recent research by Fred Travis, Ph.D., and colleagues at the Center for Brain, Consciousness, and Cognition at Maharishi University of Management shows that the longer one practices the Transcendental Meditation program, the greater the EEG coherence during mental activity in the waking state of consciousness.

The practical benefit of increasing coherence in the brain is that the mind

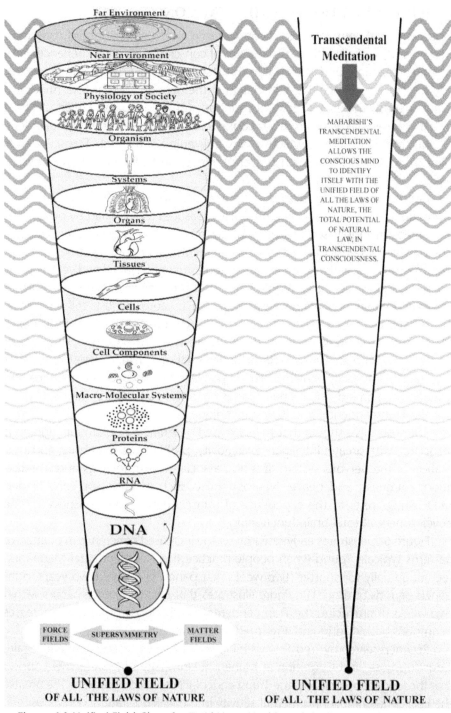

Figure 6.1 Unified Field Chart for Total Heart Health and the Transcending Process

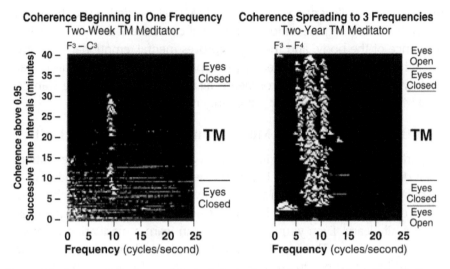

Figure 6.2. Greater Orderliness of Brain Functioning with Transcendental Meditation Practice

Source: Data from Proceedings of the San Diego Biomedical Symposium 15(1976):237–247.

and body take on a more coherent and orderly mode of functioning. Experiencing this state of restful alertness twice a day cultures the mind and body to maintain a state of greater balance. Results of a meta-analysis published in the *American Psychologist* found that Transcendental Meditation practice produces a significant increase in basal skin resistance (an indicator of reduced anxiety) and reductions in breathing rates, indicating rest and relaxation that is deeper than the kind of rest you experience by simply closing your eyes. Practicing the Transcendental Meditation technique was also found to increase the body's production of serotonin, a "rest and repair," mood-elevating hormone. These physiological changes, which correlate with a more intelligent and healthful physiology, occur and accumulate spontaneously as the mind effortlessly settles into a state of transcendental consciousness on a daily basis. These changes are the result of accessing your inner healing mechanisms, the ones that help your body to repair and restore itself. That's why people like Betty who practice the Transcendental Meditation technique begin to see the benefits almost immediately and why these benefits continue long term.

HOW TO LEARN THE TRANSCENDENTAL MEDITATION TECHNIQUE

Anyone can learn the Transcendental Meditation technique, regardless of their age, level of education, personal beliefs, or lifestyle. It's simple, natural, effortless, and easy to do. Regular practice of the Transcendental Meditation program brings about a state of deep rest to the body and the mind, eliminating the effects of stress, while it opens the mind to the greater orderliness of the unified field. In short, opening the mind to this level of consciousness restores the inner intelligence of the body, and thereby improves mental, emotional, and physical health. As we will show in later chapters, practicing this program also creates a healthy influence in your environment—all this from practicing the Transcendental Meditation technique for just twenty minutes twice a day.

What the Transcendental Meditation Technique Is and Isn't

The Transcendental Meditation technique is a simple method of meditation—it's not difficult or complicated. It is easy to learn and practice. It's natural—no manipulation or autosuggestion such as in hypnosis is required. It's effortless—no concentration or control of the mind is needed. Anyone from age ten and up can easily learn. Even younger children can learn a meditation technique specifically for them. The practice requires no physical exercises, special postures, positions, or procedures—only that you sit comfortably with eyes closed (see Figure 6.3). You can practice the Transcendental Meditation technique in the office after work, riding the subway, sitting in a plane, or in the comfort of your home. The technique is practiced for approximately twenty minutes twice daily—once in the morning before breakfast so that you can start the day with vim and energy and once again in the afternoon before dinner to eliminate the stress of the day. The benefits are often noted immediately—it doesn't take years to notice.

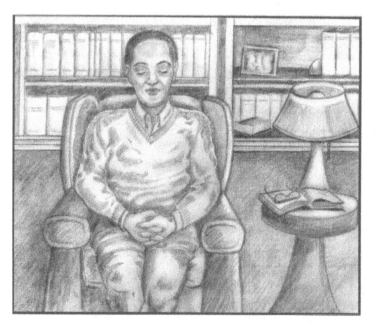

Figure 6.3.
A Gentleman
Practicing the
Transcendental
Meditation
Technique

Personal Instruction

To learn the Transcendental Meditation program requires personal instruction with a trained and certified teacher. The technique cannot be learned from books or magazines, or through cassette tapes, DVDs, or videos. There are several reasons for this.

The first reason is that each person is unique and learns at a different pace with different experiences. A qualified teacher can guide you through the steps of practice at your own pace and according to your own experiences. Teachers of the Transcendental Meditation technique undergo an intensive training program supervised by Maharishi Mahesh Yogi, the founder of the Transcendental Meditation program, where they learn how to provide instruction for all different types of people.

Another reason why it is not feasible to teach yourself the Transcendental Meditation technique by reading a book, listening to a tape, or watching a video is that these other ways cannot provide the experience of transcendental consciousness because trying to learn on your own requires effort. Effort increases mental activity while transcendental consciousness is a state of least activation of the mind. Therefore, effort and strain are polar opposites to the successful practice and beneficial effects of the Transcendental Meditation program. Also, these impersonal media can't answer all of the questions that you might have while learning the practice.

With personal instruction, you can learn how to meditate according to your needs so that you can enjoy the technique for the rest of your life, as well as enjoy all of the benefits it naturally brings. In the end, if you don't practice correctly, you won't reap the full benefits. It is only the correct, natural, and effortless practice of the Transcendental Meditation technique that brings about all the benefits shown by scientific research and clinical experience.

The Transcendental Meditation technique is taught through a seven-step course of instruction over six days. The course consists of an introductory lecture and a preparatory lecture that provide the information you need to understand the benefits and mechanics of the technique, to ask questions, and to make an informed decision. Then there is a personal interview, which is followed by four consecutive days of individual and small group instruction lasting one and a half to two hours each day.

An overview of the course structure is as follows:

- **Step 1.** Introductory Lecture: Introduces the Transcendental Meditation program and informs you of the benefits to expect from practicing this meditation technique regularly.

- **Step 2.** Preparatory Lecture: Explains the mechanics of the Transcendental

Meditation technique and how the Transcendental Meditation program works, why it's easy to learn and practice, how it's different from other meditation techniques, and the origin of the Transcendental Meditation program.

- **Step 3.** Personal Interview: An interview with a certified teacher of the Transcendental Meditation technique gives an opportunity to ask any individual questions that you may have and to make an appointment for personal instruction.

- **Step 4.** Personal Instruction: Private personal instruction in the basic steps of practice.

- **Step 5.** First Day of Checking: This is the first of a three-day series of one-and-a-half- to two-hour verification and validation meetings following personal instruction. This first day reviews the mechanics of the technique to verify and validate the correctness of your practice.

- **Step 6.** Second Day of Checking: During this second meeting, there is further instruction to verify the correctness of the practice and discuss the mechanics of how the benefits of the Transcendental Meditation program are stabilized.

- **Step 7.** Third Day of Checking: The purpose of this third day of checking is to answer questions from previous sessions and to learn about the goal of the Transcendental Meditation program—the development of your full potential and the achievement of ideal health. During this session, the long-term follow-up program is discussed. The optional follow-up program provides lifelong periodic checking of your practice and advanced lectures or topics relevant to the development of higher states of health and well-being—all available without additional charge.

To learn the Transcendental Meditation technique properly or for more details or a free introductory lecture, you may visit one of the 3,000 centers located in major cities throughout the world called Maharishi Peace Palaces or Maharishi Enlightenment Care centers. See the Resources section for a listing of some of these centers. There you can learn from a certified teacher the standard course that has been verified to produce all of the health-promoting benefits described above.

In the upcoming chapters, we will be discussing the Body Approach and the Environment Approach, each of which can synergize with the Mind Approach and help you achieve total heart health.

PART TWO

The Body Approach

❦ CHAPTER 7 ❦

Healing Your Heart Through Physiological Interventions

THE PURPOSE OF THE BODY APPROACH of the Total Heart Health program is to help create a healthy heart through physiological interventions. Like the Mind Approach, these interventions of the Body Approach help strengthen the connection of your body to its own inner intelligence. This will eliminate imbalances present in your physiology and prevent misalignments from developing in the future. These practical interventions include personalized recommendations for diet, daily and seasonal routines, exercise, and physiological purification procedures. The focus of the Body Approach is on restoring balance in the body. When this balance is achieved, your mind will also become more balanced and you will enjoy total heart health. When this happens, you won't develop heart disease, nor will you fall prey to its many risk factors.

In this chapter, we present the specific causes of heart disease and its risk factors from the perspective of the Maharishi Vedic Approach to Health, along with guidelines and questionnaires for determining what type of dosha imbalance(s), you may tend toward. (Dosha refers to the physiological principles that govern all the processes and activities of your body.) It is this imbalance that is likely to be causing your heart disease or putting you at risk. With this knowledge, you can take full advantage of the Body Approaches of the Total Heart Health program to treat and prevent these imbalances so that you may enjoy total heart health.

T he aspect of the Maharishi Vedic Approach to Health that uses physiological methods for restoring and maintaining health is also known as *Maharishi Ayurveda®*. For many centuries, the field of *Ayurveda* (literally, "the knowledge of life span") has been misunderstood and only partially practiced in the United States, and even in India, the land of its origin. As a result, its concepts and treatments have only been partially effective. Moreover, its key concepts had become fragmented and disconnected from their original source of Vedic knowledge and from the underlying unified field.

Then, in the early 1980s, Maharishi Mahesh Yogi, who brought the Transcendental Meditation® program to the West, gathered together leading Vedic physicians and scientists to evaluate the ancient science of Ayurveda. They revived the ancient knowledge and restored its original authenticity by highlighting the basis of health in the knowledge and technologies of the unified field of all the laws of nature. This allowed Maharishi Ayurveda to assume its proper role in the total health program of the Maharishi Vedic Approach to Health. Now that the true basis of the key concepts and procedures has been revived and restored so that they can more effectively enliven the body's inner intelligence, the Body Approach has become, like the Mind Approach, a core component of the Maharishi Vedic Approach to Health.

To understand how heart disease and its risk factors arise and how the Body Approach can work to prevent and treat these conditions, it is first necessary to understand a few basic principles of physiology from the ancient Vedic perspective. Two basic principles are (1) the role of fundamental physiological operators called *doshas* in Vedic terminology and (2) the role of digestion called *agni.* When the doshas are balanced and agni is strong, it allows our physiology to express the holistic value of our inner intelligence (Atma), which maintains and restores balance and health in mind and body.

DOSHAS

According to the Vedic Approach, three fundamental factors guide your physiology and influence your health. These simple but powerful factors can be explained as three governing principles of the human physiology. They are called *Vata, Pitta,* and *Kapha.* These physiological principles are called *doshas,* and they govern all the processes and activities of your body. The doshas have thousands of functions in all living things, throughout all of nature, including the human body. They can be simply thought of as mind-body operators, an operator being something that performs a particular operation or function.

John Hagelin, Ph.D., an expert in quantum physics and consciousness, and a world authority on unified field theory, views the doshas as operators that function on the most basic and powerful level of the laws of physics—the unified field. In other words, these doshas have their origin in the unified field. According to Dr. Hagelin, the doshas have a one-to-one correspondence with the fundamental operators in quantum physics called *superfields.* According to unified field theory, these three operators in nature—the gravity superfield, the gauge superfield, and the matter superfield—are fundamental categories of matter and energy close to the level of the unified field, which physicists call the *Planck scale.* Their characteristics in modern science parallel the descriptions of the three doshas provided by ancient Vedic scientists. The doshas, then, like their associated superfields, are at the basis of the physical world including the human physiology, with their roots in the nonmaterial quantum level of the unified field.

Figure 7.1 illustrates the correspondence between the fundamental laws of nature described by quantum physics and the doshas described by ancient Vedic science.

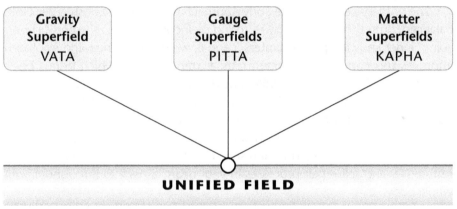

Figure 7.1. Doshas and Quantum Physics

Understanding how the doshas operate and generate all levels of physiology—from the subtlest levels of the unified field to acting as mind-body operators in the human physiology—helps explain their importance in the Maharishi Vedic Approach to Health. Because the doshas operate at the most basic level of the body, at the point where the unified field first becomes expressed as matter, imbalances in the doshas are at the root cause of disease. While the physiologies of all individuals are generated from a combination of the three doshas, the exact proportion of each dosha differs from individual to individual. It follows that the imbalances that arise in each of us will be different, even though the end result—for example, heart disease—may be similar. This understanding can then be used to individualize treatment for imbalances and diseases, including heart disease.

The understanding that it is essential to address the specific dosha or quantum mechanical imbalances in each person does not exist in modern medicine, which works only at more gross levels of the physiology. In contrast, the Maharishi Vedic Approach to Health, with its understanding of the primordial role of the doshas, works on a more subtle or quantum mechanical level of physiology, one that guides the material level of physiology that we see and touch with our ordinary senses.

Imbalances can arise in an individual when one or more doshas become excessive or aggravated. The Body Approach diagnoses and treats imbalances that are present in Vata, Pitta, and Kapha doshas and their subgroups. An imbalance in the doshas is a sign of a disruption in the flow of the body's inner intelligence from the unified field. Under normal conditions where the doshas are in balance, this flow is responsible for the proper functioning of all aspects of the body's physiology.

The primary purpose of the Body Approach is to bring the doshas back into balanced, orderly functioning by restoring their connection to the body's reservoir of inner knowledge. In Chapters 5 and 6, we saw how the Mind Approach improves this connection through regular transcending, which brings one's awareness to the level of the unified field. The Body Approach also improves this connection but does so through physiological practices that balance the doshas. Restoring the proper functioning of the doshas, which are basic expressions of biological intelligence, is the physical equivalent to enlivening the body's inner intelligence. This all results in the promotion of natural-healing, restorative, and self-repair processes in your heart, as well as throughout your whole body.

Basic Functions of the Doshas

While the doshas are responsible for thousands of specific actions in the body, each dosha has a main physiological area. And further, because the body and mind are intimately connected with each other, the physiological effects of the doshas also express themselves in the qualities of thoughts, emotions, and behavior in a person. The following is a summary of the basic functions of the doshas:

- **Vata** is responsible for regulating *movement.* This includes the heartbeat; movement of blood through the tissues; exchange of air, food, and water in each cell; transmission of nerve impulses; and signals that urge cells to operate. It is also responsible for thinking.

- **Pitta** is responsible for regulating *transformation* (that is, metabolism), including energy production, and heat. This also includes digestion and the metabolism of food, air, and water by the cells.

- **Kapha** is responsible for regulating *structure.* This includes building cells and tissues and regulating the amount of water and fat in the cells and tissues.

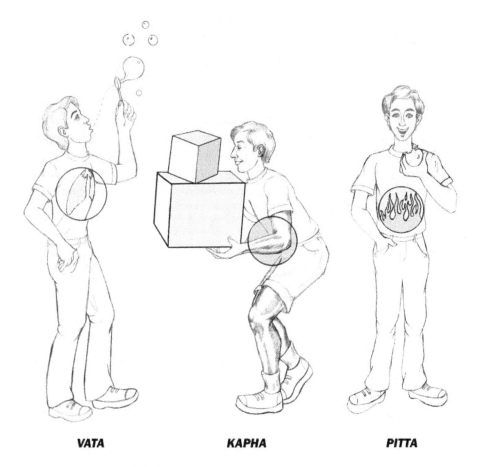

VATA   KAPHA   PITTA

Figure 7.2. Functions of the Doshas

Primary Qualities of the Dosha

All three doshas are present in varying combinations in the mind and body, in all living things, and in all of nature. Each of us is a mixture of Vata, Pitta, and Kapha, although, as we will discuss later, one dosha will usually be most promi-nent in our mind-body type. More important for our purposes here, this pre-dominant dosha will usually be more out of balance than the others. The predominant imbalanced dosha will typically be the primary cause of your risk factors and predisposition to heart disease. Therefore, in the Body Approach of the Total Heart Health program we will focus our attention and treatments on your predominant imbalanced dosha.

Following are the primary qualities associated with each dosha:

• **Vata** is quick, light, cold, and dry. People dominated by Vata are quick acting and thinking; they like change; they can be restless and anxious, and their bodies are thin and lean. They are inclined to get very enthusiastic about new things but have trouble sticking to them. They tend toward creative or intellectual pursuits.

- **Pitta** is hot, sharp, acidic, and slightly oily. People dominated by Pitta seem to have an inner fire with forceful actions and thinking. They have abundant drive, but tend to get irritated under pressure. Their bodies are medium in height, weight, and physical strength. Their complexion is generally fair or reddish. They tend to have strong digestions and good appetites and don't like missing a meal. They gravitate toward order and perfection in their lives and make good organizers. They can be very focused and intense, and are passionate by nature.

- **Kapha** is heavy, oily, slow, cold, steady, solid, and dull. People dominated by Kapha are steady, methodical, and calm. Their bodies are often heavy-set, tending to overweight. They are strong, with great physical stamina and endurance, but can also tend toward lethargy. Their skin is usually soft and oily and they have large lustrous eyes and thick hair. On the whole, they are slower in nature, slower in digesting food, slower in taking in information, and slower in speech. They may be generally sweet natured and emotionally stable. We think of them as being grounded or earthy.

In the Total Heart Health program, we take into account a person's unique psychophysiological makeup in the form of dosha balance. This allows one to precisely tailor the intervention to the specific needs of the individual, whether it be for prevention or treatment.

For example, consider obesity, one of the risk factors for heart disease, and three overweight people: Georgia, Dianne, and Tom. Georgia is frequently anxious, a fast talker, and eats quickly. She exhibits a dominance of Vata qualities. Dianne is ruddy complexioned, hot-tempered, and prone to heartburn with a dominance of Pitta qualities. Tom is slow and often lethargic, exhibiting a dominance of Kapha qualities. All three are overweight but the underlying cause of their obesity is fundamentally different. Therefore, the treatment and preventive measures for restoring ideal weight will be different for each because, if it is going to be effective, the therapeutic program must match the type of imbalance in the individual.

It's the same with heart disease and its other major risk factors. The Maharishi Vedic Approach to Health considers the individual's type of dosha imbalance to determine the course of treatment and prevention. Each person will need to determine his or her predominant imbalanced dosha, and keep it in

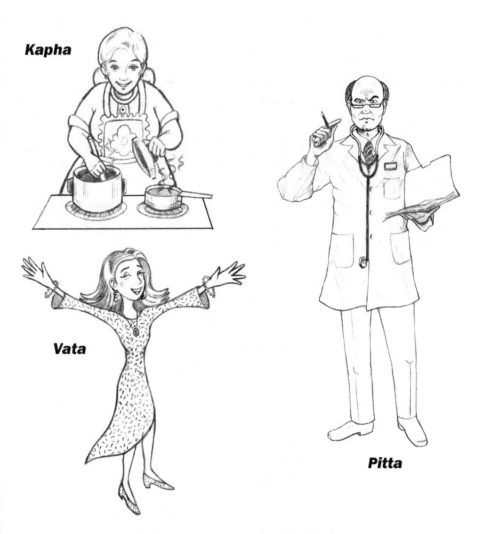

Figure 7.3. Qualities of the Doshas

mind in order to implement the Total Heart Health program later. Identifying your predominant dosha type can be done by filling out the questionnaires later in this chapter.

How the Doshas Are Expressed

All three doshas are involved in the creation of both health and disease. When the three doshas are in balance, the mind and body are in balance and, in turn, you experience good health and well-being. On the other hand, when the doshas are out of balance, meaning that there is an excess of one or more doshas, the initial conditions have been established for development of disease. Following are the typical physical and mental traits characteristic of each dosha when all three are properly functioning:

- **When Vata is in balance, you can expect:** Mental alertness, proper formation of body tissues, normal elimination, strong immunity, sound sleep, and a sense of exhilaration.

- **When Pitta is in balance, you can expect:** Normal body heat and thirst, strong digestion, sharp intellect, lustrous complexion, courage, and contentment.

- **When Kapha is in balance, you can expect:** Excellent muscular strength, strong immunity, affection, generosity, confidence, dignity, normal joint activity, vitality, and a stable mind.

Each dosha has five subdivisions, or subdoshas. Each subdosha has a different responsibility within the framework of its major dosha. This partitioning not only provides a division of labor, but it also helps make diagnosis and treatment of a dosha imbalance more accurate. For example, one important subdosha of Vata is called *Prana Vata,* which is located in the heart, upper chest, and head. Prana Vata regulates the beating of the heart, and the movement of breath and nerve impulses, and, as such, it influences every function of the body.

One important subdosha of Pitta is called *Sadhaka Pitta,* which is located in the heart. It regulates the heart's connection to the brain and emotions. *Avalambaka Kapha* gives structure and stability to the heart. Knowing some information about the subdoshas can help you to better understand the state of balance within you, and why you might have the cardiovascular symptoms you have.

Table 7.1 describes the specific functions of the fifteen subdoshas and the most common symptoms that occur when their balance is disturbed.

Doshas and their subdoshas can be thrown out of balance by diet or behavior that is inappropriate for your mind-body type. The lifestyle factors with the greatest potential to aggravate each dosha are listed below.

Lifestyle Factors That Aggravate Vata

- Cold foods and drinks
- Cold, dry, windy weather
- Constant multitasking
- Eating at a different time every day

TABLE 7.1. THE DOSHAS AND THEIR SUBDOSHAS

Subdoshas Govern . . .	Characteristic Symptoms of Subdosha Imbalance
Vata	
Prana Vata: the senses, respiratory system, creative thinking, reasoning, enthusiasm	Prana Vata: worries, overactive mind, sleep problems, difficulty breathing
Udana Vata: quality of voice, memory, movements of thought	Udana Vata: dry coughs, sore throats, earaches, general fatigue
Samana Vata: movement of food through the digestive tract	Samana Vata: slow or rapid digestion, gas, intestinal cramps, poor assimilation, weak tissues
Apana Vata: movement through the digestive system, elimination of wastes, sexual function	Apana Vata: intestinal cramps, menstrual problems, lower back pain, irregularity, diarrhea, constipation, gas
Vyana Vata: blood flow, heart rhythm, perspiration, sense of touch	Vyana Vata: nervousness, shakiness, poor blood flow, coldness, high blood pressure
Pitta	
Pachaka Pitta: digestion, assimilation metabolism for healthy nutrients and tissues	Pachaka Pitta: acid stomach
Ranjaka Pitta: healthy, toxin-free blood	Ranjaka Pitta: early graying of hair, anger, toxins in the blood
Sadhaka Pitta: desire, drive, decisiveness, spirituality	Sadhaka Pitta: demanding, perfectionist, workaholic
Alochaka Pitta: functioning of the eyes	Alochaka Pitta: blood shot eyes, poor vision
Bhrajaka Pitta: healthy glow of skin	Bhrajaka Pitta: skin rashes, acne
Kapha	
Kledaka Kapha: moisture of the stomach lining	Kledaka Kapha: impaired digestion, poor absorption
Avalambaka Kapha: protects the heart, strong muscles, healthy lungs	Avalambaka Kapha: lethargy, respiratory problems, lower back pain
Bhodaka Kapha: sense of taste (vital for good digestion)	Bhodaka Kapha: poor sense of taste, food cravings from lack of fulfillment
Shleshaka Kapha: lubrication of the joints, softness and suppleness of skin	Shleshaka Kapha: weight gain, oily skin, loose or painful joints
Tarpaka Kapha: moisture for nose, mouth, eyes, and brain	Tarpaka Kapha: sinus congestion, poor sense of smell

- Eating too fast
- Eating too much of light, dry, and pungent foods
- Eating while in the car
- Eating while standing up
- Eating while working or talking on the phone
- Feeling pressured on the job or at home
- Insomnia
- Rushing around
- Skipping meals
- Staying awake after 10:00 P.M.
- Too much mental work
- Too much TV, especially at night
- Working at night

Lifestyle Factors That Aggravate Pitta

- Associating with people who are habitually angry or critical
- Eating foods that are made with chemicals, preservatives, or were grown with chemical fertilizers
- Eating in a hurry
- Eating too much spicy, salty, and sour foods
- Eating while distracted
- Exposure to emotional stress
- Exposure to hot weather
- Overexerting or exercising in the hot sun
- Pressured situations at work or at home
- Skipping or delaying meals
- Staying awake after 10:00 P.M.

Lifestyle Factors That Aggravate Kapha

- Cold foods and drinks
- Cool, wet weather
- Eating leftovers, packaged foods, processed foods, fast foods

- Eating while standing up
- Eating foods that are too rich and high in fat
- Eating foods that are too sweet, sour, or salty
- Lack of mental stimulation
- Not exercising
- Sleeping during the day
- Waking after 6:00 A.M.
- Snacking before the previous meal is digested

THE ROLE OF DIGESTION AND AGNI

The second fundamental principle that sets the Maharishi Vedic Approach to Health apart from conventional medicine is that it considers a strong digestion to be essential for health. *Agni* is the process and power of digestion, and it is sometimes translated as fire. It has a major role in maintaining health and preventing heart disease.

In the body, agni metabolizes food into nutrients that you use and assimilate. This occurs not only in the gastrointestinal tract but also in each and every cell. Proper digestion of food is important for two reasons: one, food supplies the body with the raw materials it needs to build and renew itself daily; and two, improper digestion of the nutrients in food leads to incompletely digested food residues, or toxins called *ama,* that accumulate and cause dosha imbalance and disease. In the body, agni is found especially in the digestive juices in the stomach and intestines. A strong digestion supports proper functioning of the doshas while a weak digestion can disturb any or all of the doshas.

Shrotas

Shrotas are the innumerable channels of communication throughout the body. Some shrotas are visible to the human eye, appearing as arteries, veins, tear ducts, the lymph system, and others. Other shrotas are less visible. For example, each cell is surrounded by a cell membrane that contains thousands of tiny channels that transport nutrients into the cells and waste products out of them. This is important to the overall process of digestion.

Each shrota is designed to function as a channel for the movement of one or more doshas throughout the body. If a shrota is disrupted or becomes blocked, such as in a clogged coronary artery, its essential tasks are hindered. A narrowed or blocked coronary artery, for example, does not allow for a sufficient blood supply to reach the heart muscle. This blocked shrota in the heart is the structural basis of coronary heart disease.

Dhatus

During digestion, food is broken down into subsidiary nutrients that are metabolized into the body's main tissues. The Maharishi Vedic Approach to Health calls these tissues *dhatus*. Proper formation of the dhatus requires a healthy digestion and metabolism. Any block in the process of digestion will show up as a weakness in a tissue and in all the tissues that derive from it. This also leads to dosha imbalance and eventually to disease.

Dhatus are formed in a specific sequence. Their formation begins with Rasa, followed by Rakta, Mamsa, Meda, Asthi, Majja, and ends with Shukra. Dhatus approximately correspond to the modern physiological concept of tissues. This correlation of dhatus and tissues is summarized as follows:

- **Rasa:** Plasma, nutrient fluids

- **Rakta:** Blood cells, hemoglobin

- **Mamsa:** Muscle

- **Meda:** Fat, adipose tissue

- **Asthi:** Bone

- **Majja:** Bone marrow, central nervous system tissue

- **Shukra:** Reproductive tissue

Ama: The Result of Poor Digestion

When agni or digestion is poor and the doshas are out of balance, the body produces a toxic substance called *ama*. This substance is the remains of undigested or improperly digested food, and it causes havoc throughout the body. Ama blocks the flow in the body's essential channels, or shrotas, impeding the flow of intelligence, or worse, it circulates throughout the body's tissues and organs, aggravating the doshas and disturbing the dhatus.

Suffice it to say for now that the combination of weak digestion, ama, clogged shrotas, and dosha imbalance can arise not only from poor diet, but also from many other lifestyle behaviors such as those listed earlier that aggravate the dosha. Ultimately, the dosha imbalance becomes great enough that it causes symptoms that we recognize as part of a disease. Because this villain (ama) is the harbinger of heart disease and other chronic disorders, physiological recommendations of the Maharishi Vedic Approach to Health aim at reducing and eliminating ama as a key goal.

Figure 7.4 illustrates the path to heart disease and how all these physiological elements fit together to cause heart disease from the traditional viewpoint of Vedic physiology. In this scheme, any one of the three doshas can become aggravated. This imbalance, together with improper digestion or agni, leads to imbalance at the tissue or dhatus level, and results, for example, in high cholesterol. The aggravated tissue then blocks the corresponding channel or shrota and leads to atherosclerosis of the arteries in the heart.

| Dosha aggravated | + | Agni aggravated (too weak, strong, or irregular) | → | Dhatu aggravated | → | Shrotas blocked (atherosclerosis) |

Figure 7.4. The Path to Heart Disease from the Viewpoint of Vedic Physiology

Ojas and Good Health

When your digestion is strong, functioning properly, and extracting the nutrients it needs, your body produces a health-promoting substance called *ojas.* Ojas circulates throughout the body and is responsible for the body's strength and resilience. Having sufficient amounts of ojas moving freely through the mind and body is like wearing a protective shield. It keeps the doshas balanced and it increases resistance to influences that cause disease. When the production of ojas decreases, the body weakens and becomes more susceptible to disease. Moderate and healthy eating and lifestyle habits promote the production of ojas, while eating the wrong foods and following an unhealthy lifestyle destroy it. The Body Approach seeks to promote the production of ojas for all around good health.

Now that you have been introduced to the key physiological concepts involved in the Body Approach of the Total Heart Health program, we can begin to view the causes of heart disease and its risk factors from a new perspective. The remainder of this chapter discusses some of the key tools you can use to determine where the root of your heart disease may be.

DIAGNOSING IMBALANCES IN YOUR DOSHAS

The Total Heart Health program uses a variety of methods to accurately diagnose the status of your health. One simple technique used to determine imbalances is called *pulse diagnosis,* or *nadi vigyan.* Unlike typical high-tech tests used by conventional medicine that may or may not pinpoint the basis of your discomfort, pain, or disease, pulse diagnosis is reliable and noninvasively detects underlying physiological tendencies and patterns. It gives a person insight into dosha imbalances that are causing his or her symptoms and disease. A pulse reading gives feedback not only on your general state of health and dosha tendencies, but also gives accurate feedback regarding specific imbalances in the doshas and subdoshas that could lead to, or have led to, disease. Moreover, it provides information on the condition of the agni, shrotas, dhatus, and the presence of ama.

To perform pulse diagnosis, a physician or practitioner of the Vedic approach places three fingers on the radial artery at the wrist (see Figure 7.5). When placed properly, and with the correct amount of pressure, the first (index) finger feels the Vata pulse; the second (middle) finger feels the Pitta pulse; the third (ring) finger feels the Kapha pulse. From the condition of the pulse—which includes a large number of characteristics—the expert can evaluate the status of your body systems. Since disease begins as subtle dosha imbalances, long before symptoms develop, pulse diagnosis allows the Maharishi Vedic Approach to Health practitioner to diagnosis a disease much earlier than a conventional doctor can, who relies on overt symptoms. This helps to avert disease at a very early stage, before symptoms and even before laboratory tests show abnormalities.

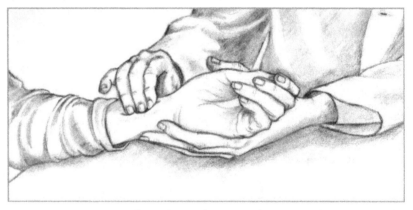

Figure 7.5. Pulse Diagnosis

Self-Pulse Diagnosis

Proficiency in using pulse diagnosis comes with practice but the basics can be learned by anyone. As a matter of fact, facilities and schools that teach courses on the Maharishi Vedic Approach to Health offer self-pulse diagnosis training so that you can easily detect your daily health needs by feeling your own pulse (see the Resources section). Checking your pulse regularly not only alerts you to imbalances that may be addressed through simple adjustment in diet, routine, or behavior, but also the procedure has a soothing and restorative effect of its own, presumably through the act of putting one's attention on the body in a very subtle way.

Other Diagnostic Tools

In addition to pulse diagnosis, the Maharishi Vedic Approach to Health uses several other diagnostic tools to determine dosha imbalances and home in on the causes of heart disease, or any type of illness. Two of these tools are the medical interview and physical examination, in which the physician or practitioner gathers information about an individual's behavioral and lifestyle tendencies. Another tool is the self-assessment questionnaire that is used to help determine the predominant dosha that is out of balance. This is the most likely dosha that is causing your predisposition to heart disease.

This brings out another difference between the Maharishi Vedic Approach to Health and modern medicine. The Total Heart Health program emphasizes the ability of the individual to care for his or her own health through simple and easy-to-use diagnostic tools. The following questionnaires reprinted with permission from Maharishi Ayurveda Products International (MAPI) will help you to determine your predominant imbalanced dosha. You can use the results of this questionnaire to guide your choices of dosha-specific recommendations in later chapters in Part Two. For a more sophisticated and complete diagnosis, consult your Maharishi Vedic Approach to Health physician or practitioner (see the Resources section).

Questionnaire 1: Do You Need to Balance Vata Dosha?

Answer the following questions to determine if you need to balance Vata dosha:

1. Is your skin dry, rough, thin?

2. Are you underweight?

3. Is your mind constantly in a whirl?

4. Do you worry incessantly?

5. Are you constantly agitated or restless?

6. Do you experience constipation?

7. Do you suffer from insomnia?

8. Do you suffer from vaginal dryness?

9. Do you have spells of forgetfulness?

10. Do you experience discomfort in the joints?

11. Are you easily fatigued?

If you answered yes to *six* or more of these questions, you need to pacify (decrease) Vata dosha. Diet, exercise, and daily and seasonal routine recommendations are given in the next chapters to help you balance Vata-type heart disease or risk factors.

Questionnaire 2: Do You Need to Balance Pitta Dosha?

Answer the following questions to determine if you need to balance Pitta dosha:

1. Do you tend to be demanding or critical?

2. Are you often frustrated, angry, or intense?

3. Is your skin ruddy and prone to rashes and eruptions?

4. Are you often irritable or impatient?

5. Is your hair prematurely gray or thinning?

6. Do you wake up in the early hours and find it difficult to fall asleep again?

7. Do you feel discomfort in hot weather?

8. Are you a perfectionist?

9. Do you experience hot flashes?

10. Do you have excess stomach acid?

11. Do you experience loose bowel movements?

If you answered yes to *six* or more of these questions, you need to pacify Pitta dosha. Dietary, exercise, daily and seasonal routine recommendations are given in the next chapters to help balance Pitta-type heart disease or risk factors.

Questionnaire 3: Do You Need to Balance Kapha Dosha?

Answer the following questions to determine if you need to balance Kapha dosha:

1. Do you tend to be overweight?

2. Are you often oversettled or lethargic?

3. Do you have sinus problems?

4. Do you sleep long hours yet wake up unrefreshed?

5. Are your skin and hair oily?

6. Are you possessive or overly attached (to things or people)?

7. Are you uncomfortable in cold weather?

8. Do you feel lazy, complacent?

9. Do you experience bloating, water retention?

10. Do you feel stiff and heavy, especially in the morning?

11. Do you experience congestion?

If you answered yes to *six* or more of these questions, you need to pacify Kapha dosha. Dietary, exercise, daily and seasonal routine recommendations are given in the next chapters to help balance Kapha-type heart disease or risk factors.

If your score indicates that you need to pacify two doshas, follow recommendations for the highest scoring dosha first. Then you may retake the questionnaire after two to three months and redetermine your dosha balance. If what had been the highest scoring dosha has decreased (score less than 6), then readjust your diet and routine to the new predominant dosha type.

Now that you have determined which doshas are out of balance and are likely to be contributing to your heart disease or to its risk factors, you can use this valuable information as the basis for applying the specific guidelines in the following chapters for bringing Vatta, Pitta, and Kapha back to their proper functioning. Simple changes in your diet and daily routines can bring dramatic results, as the lost connection between your body and its own inner intelligence is reunited. As noted earlier, when possible, it is helpful to consult with a the Maharishi Vedic physician or practitioner. Also, we always recommend that you consult with your doctor as you undertake your new prevention-oriented program.

♥ CHAPTER 8 ♥

Diet for a Healthy Heart: Basic Principles for Your Mind-Body Type

IN BOTH MODERN MEDICINE AND THE MAHARISHI VEDIC Approach to Health, diet plays a key role in the prevention and treatment of heart disease. However, in the Total Heart Health program, diet involves not only what you eat, but also how you eat, digest, and metabolize food. Even how the food is prepared and when and how it is consumed have an influence on your health. And most important, as in all the Total Heart Health approaches, the ultimate purpose of diet and digestion is to restore the body's own healing potential by waking up the storehouse of biological intelligence deep within every cell.

Increasing the flow of intelligence allows the body's own natural healing mechanisms to work to their fullest potential, which, in turn, creates balanced functioning in the physiological processes of your cardiovascular system and in the whole body. Whether we call this state one of balanced doshas or balanced physiology, it is the basis for the Body Approach to total heart health. In this chapter, we cover the basics of the program's heart-healthy diet and digestion recommendations for balancing your doshas and for prevention and treatment of heart disease and its risk factors.

In the fifteen years since he retired as a machine mechanic, Ken, age seventy-nine, had suffered from hypertension, high cholesterol, and atherosclerosis. After bypass surgery, he tried unsuccessfully to lose weight and lower his cholesterol and blood pressure. Then, last year, his doctor encouraged him to start a Maharishi Vedic Approach to Health routine that included practicing the Transcendental Meditation program, eating a customized vegetarian diet to balance his doshas, and taking Vedic healthcare herbal supplements to lower his blood pressure and his cholesterol. After three months on his new routine,

Ken was a new man. "I wish I would have started this fifteen years ago," he says. "I've lost almost thirty pounds in three months. My cholesterol is way down and my blood pressure is 120/67."

At first the new routine required some adjustments for Ken, but he noticed improvements so quickly that he was eager to continue. The longer he stuck with the program, the more benefits he gained. "Now my cholesterol is below 120 and my doctor has practically taken me off my cholesterol medication. I'm going to see if I can go off it all together," says Ken. "My blood pressure has been steadily going down. I can walk now without having to stop and rest. I'm really pleased with it."

THE NATURE OF FOOD

It has been said you are what you eat. This is literally true as food provides the molecules that make up the structure of your body. Food also contains and provides energy and key nutrients required for specific body functions such as movement and metabolism. According to the traditional Vedic approach to health, however, food is also medicine. Or at least it has the potential to be, if you eat right. This is brought out in an old proverb from one of the ancient Vedic texts, "without proper diet, medicine is of no use. With proper diet, medicine is of no need."

The reason is that food can be used to balance your doshas, and when your doshas are balanced, you enjoy better physical and mental health. This is so because food is made from the same laws of physics, chemistry, and biology as the human physiology. These laws of nature are contained as "packets of intelligence" in the food. If your diet is proper for you and your physiology, these packets of intelligence will restore the intelligence in your body as a whole and in your heart and blood vessels specifically. This is different from modern medicine's concept of minimum daily requirements of vitamins, minerals, proteins, carbohydrates, and fats. These provide some building blocks for structures in the workings of your body, but from nature's point of view, diet has the potential to restore the details of the blueprint that creates your body.

As you learned in the previous chapter, heart disease and its risk factors have been described in the ancient Vedic literature as the result of deep-rooted disturbances in the functioning of the doshas. Doshas are the basic quantum mechanical operators within the human physiology. Now that you have estimated which dosha is primarily aggravated (generally due to too much of it), a specific diet can help rebalance it. And once imbalances and disease are eliminated, diet is an efficient way to keep the doshas in balance for prevention.

This approach goes beyond avoiding a few unhealthy types of foods, foods that are high in cholesterol or saturated fats, for example. It even goes beyond eating whole grains, vegetables, and fruits. It is an approach in which your entire diet is customized to your unique physiological type and in this way helps to make your heart healthier and you happier. Like learning anything new, it may take a little time to become familiar with the theory and practice; but you should find, like Ken did, that you will begin to feel better, which will make it so much easier to stick with your new diet plan.

KEY PRINCIPLES OF THE PROGRAM'S HEART-HEALTHY DIETS

When the ancient Vedic texts state that food is medicine, it means that each type of food has well-defined physiological effects, which can be used to restore proper physiological functioning. Two aspects of food that are particularly important are quality and taste. The diet should also contain all six tastes, but the proportions of each taste taken should be according to your individual dosha balance. Let's consider each of these aspects briefly.

Follow a Vegetarian Diet

From the traditional viewpoint of the Vedic approach, a lacto-vegetarian diet is the healthiest diet for your heart. Lacto-vegetarian diets include no meat, chicken, fish, or eggs, but do include dairy products. In fact, medical research worldwide has shown that people who eat vegetarian diets have a significantly lower incidence of heart disease than meat-eaters. Consider these scientific reports:

- Vegetarians suffer significantly lower death rates from heart disease than nonvegetarians. In a British study of vegetarians and nonvegetarians among 78,000 individuals, mortality from heart disease was 57 percent lower in vegetarians than in the general population and 18 percent lower than among nonvegetarians following an otherwise healthy lifestyle.

- A study of 25,000 vegetarian Seventh-Day Adventists documented a link between meat consumption and heart disease. Among middle-aged men, those who ate meat daily were three times more likely to die from heart disease than those who did not eat meat.

- Results from an eleven-year study of almost 2,000 German vegetarians found death from cardiovascular disease to be 61 percent lower in male vegetarians and 44 percent lower in female vegetarians than in the general population.

Vedic health care recommends eating a vegetarian diet, not only because it is lower in saturated fats, cholesterol, and "empty calories" found in processed and refined foods, but also because it is lighter and easier to digest. In traditional Vedic terminology, this creates fewer impurities (ama) in the system whereas meat is more difficult to digest and metabolize and, along with the high cholesterol and fat content, creates more ama. From this perspective, consumption of meat tends to clog a person's shrotas, weaken digestion, and produce ama, or toxins, which can spread to other parts of the body, particularly to your arteries. This leads to a buildup of fatty plaque that blocks your life-giving coronary arteries.

Following a lacto-vegetarian diet is a goal to aim for, but many individuals may want to do this gradually. Since the least heart-healthy meat is considered to be red meat, you might include poultry and fish but not red meat in your diet, if desired, according to the recommendations given later. An example of a well-known diet that is high in fruits and vegetables and low in meat is the Mediterranean diet. Experts in heart disease often recommend it because scientific research has shown that people who consume this type of diet have reduced rates of heart disease and tend to live longer. In one well-known study, among 1,507 men and 832 women aged seventy to ninety years, adhering to a Mediterranean diet was associated with a more than 50 percent lower rate of mortality from coronary heart disease and other cardiovascular diseases.

Eat Fresh, Organically Grown Food

For maximum nutritional value and digestibility, eat food that has been organically grown without the use of harmful chemicals found in pesticides, herbicides, and certain fertilizers. Favor food that is freshly prepared. Avoid leftovers, canned and frozen foods, and processed and pre-prepared foods. Also, avoid produce grown from genetically modified plants.

The process of genetically modifying food is a disturbing trend in modern agriculture. Some seed producers manipulate the characteristics of a plant using genetic engineering technologies (cloning animals is another example of genetic engineering). The intent is to increase crop production, making them cheaper to grow and market. Foods that are genetically modified or are derived from genetically modified organisms (GMO) are not recommended by the Maharishi Vedic Approach to Health. While natural or organic non-GMO foods have been shown over thousands of years to be safe to eat, the effects of growing and eating GMO foods have not been adequately tested. In his book *Genetic Engineering: The Hazards* noted molecular biologist and former National Institutes of Health scientist John Fagan, Ph.D., points out that although genetic engineers can alter DNA with reasonable precision, they cannot fully and reliably predict the biological effects of these alterations. The list of potential hazards associated with producing GMO foods includes toxic reactions and side effects, creation of new diseases, genetic pollution (introduction of toxic DNA elements into the agricultural gene pool), disruption of soil ecology, and disruption of the ecosystem. Also, growing genetically modified crops requires greater use of toxic, carcinogenic, and mutagenic agricultural chemicals, which contributes to water pollution and, in turn, to increased incidences of cancer, birth defects, and other illnesses.

Look for a "certified organic" label on foods and food products that specifically states "non-genetically modified" (often abbreviated as "NON-GMO"). This label assures you that the food is free of genetically altered organisms, growth-enhancing chemicals, harmful additives, and preservatives, and is safe for eating.

The way your food is grown can have a powerful influence on the quality and the vitality of the food. Our perspective is that foods grown according to the principles and techniques of Maharishi Vedic Organic Agriculture℠ are the healthiest foods you can eat. This is because Maharishi Vedic farming practices, in keeping with the restoration of this ancient system of Vedic agriculture, adhere to the most rigorous certification standards for organic food and go well beyond even contemporary organic standards.

Vedic agriculture recognizes the fundamental link between man and nature and seeks to enhance that relationship in its farming practices. The practices of Maharishi Vedic Organic Agriculture include applying Vedic sounds and music in the fields to enliven the intelligence and vitality within the plants and to enhance balance in the surrounding environment. (See Chapter 14 for details on Vedic sound programs.) When you consume such foods, you benefit from the enlivened biological intelligence in the food itself. Organic foods grown according to Vedic standards are becoming more readily available to consumers. (See the Resources section for further information.)

Incorporate the "Six Tastes" into Each Meal

Unlike the U.S. Department of Agriculture's Food Guide Pyramid that classifies foods according to conventional food groups such as fruits, vegetables, dairy, and grains, or by biochemical category such as rich in proteins, carbohydrates, and fats, the Maharishi Vedic Approach to Health groups foods according to how they affect the doshas in the body. This includes their qualities, such as hot/cold, oily/dry, heavy/light (see Chapter 7), and their tastes, which we'll talk about next.

First mention of the six tastes is found in the ancient Vedic texts. Each taste was distinct from the others and was noted to produce specific physiological effects on the body. The six tastes are sweet, sour, salty, pungent (spicy, hot), bitter, and astringent. Most foods contain several tastes, but one taste always dominates. Strategically incorporating foods with these tastes into your diet allows you to selectively affect the balance of the doshas in your body. In turn, this allows you to prevent or ameliorate imbalances, which helps prevent future disease.

Interestingly, diets based on these principles are also nutritionally balanced according to the criteria of modern medicine. When you eat a diet that is balanced according to the six tastes and other principles given in this and upcoming chapters in Part Two, you will naturally consume a healthful balance of proteins, carbohydrates, healthy fats, vitamins, and minerals.

How do tastes correspond to different types of physiological effects? It's a way of gauging the effects of foods. Using food for this purpose is different from modern diets, where taste is merely for aesthetics. In the Maharishi Vedic Approach to Health, taste serves as a window into the quantum mechanical effects of food on the body. (Remember our discussion in Chapter 4 on the basic forces of nature where all things are connected on the quantum level?) In other words, a food's taste tells you how it will affect your doshas. Each taste tells you how the food may be used to restore balance in your body, thereby providing for its deepest needs.

Following are examples of foods found in each of the six taste groups. The list is based on the predominant taste of each food item and groups the foods according to their effects on the doshas as described next:

- **Sweet:** Sugar, honey, milk, butter, bread, grains, pasta, rice, sweet ripe fruits, and juicy vegetables such as summer squash

- **Sour:** Yogurt, cheeses, tofu, and lemon

- **Salty:** Table salt, soy sauce, and foods prepared with salt (pretzels, potato chips, and others)

- **Pungent:** Spices (cayenne, chili peppers, cumin, ginger, and black pepper) and foods such as radishes and mustard greens

- **Bitter:** Greens such as endive and parsley, leafy green vegetables such as chard and kale, sprouts

- **Astringent:** Beans and legumes (including lentils), pomegranates, persimmons, cabbage, cauliflower, broccoli, and spinach

Initially, you may need to refer to this list (and the other dietary information in this book) to favor foods that correct your predominant dosha imbalance. Over time, though, by paying attention to the experiences you have when you eat certain foods, you will naturally start to favor foods that are balancing for you. In this chapter, we give many examples of foods that correspond to each taste and dosha effect. (For a more extensive list of specific foods and their effects on each dosha, see the MAPI website. This web address can be found in the Resources section.)

You decrease or pacify a dosha by eating foods whose predominant tastes are opposite to the characteristics of the dosha. You increase a dosha (and aggravate it) and risk causing an imbalance by eating foods whose predominant tastes are similar to the characteristics of the dosha. In other words, "like increases like" and "opposites decrease each other." So you can decrease or pacify a target dosha by consuming foods with tastes that have opposite effects. (See Table 8.1.)

You can see from Table 8.1 that certain tastes increase certain doshas while other tastes pacify them. For example, Vata dosha is decreased by sweet, sour, and salty foods, while Kapha dosha is increased by the same three tastes; the converse is true for pungent, bitter, and astringent tastes (they decrease Kapha and increase Vata). Pitta dosha is decreased by sweet, bitter, and astringent tastes; salt, sour, and pungent foods aggravate Pitta dosha that is already sharp and hot.

TABLE 8.1. HOW TO USE THE SIX TASTES TO HELP RESTORE DOSHA BALANCE	
EFFECT	TASTES TO FAVOR
Decrease Vata	Sweet, sour, salty
Increase Vata	Pungent, bitter, astringent
Decrease Pitta	Sweet, bitter, astringent
Increase Pitta	Pungent, sour, salty
Decrease Kapha	Pungent bitter, astringent
Increase Kapha	Sweet, sour, salty

These principles are incorporated into the recommendations in the tables later in this chapter. The same principle—that like increases like—holds true for the qualities of foods. For example, Vata dosha is described as being quick, light, cold, and dry. Therefore, foods that are light, cold, and dry will increase (aggravate) Vata while foods that are heavier, warm, and unctuous will decrease (pacify) Vata.

Of course, a balanced meal should include all six tastes. If you include certain tastes to pacify a dosha imbalance, you should also include the other tastes to some degree in your meal to ensure physiological balance. This should not be hard to accomplish, and with time, you will see that choosing the right tastes in the right amounts for your mind-body type comes more easily. Animals instinctually know what foods to eat (they don't read labels very well) and so do human babies (studies have shown that if given the choice to eat many different foods, babies will eat a nourishing diet). So that you won't have to rely totally on instinct just yet, the tables in this chapter provide you with expert advice on what foods and tastes to eat if you are trying to prevent or treat heart disease.

BALANCING YOUR DOSHAS WITH DIET

Now that we have discussed the fundamental principles of the program's heart-healthy diets, let's talk about the specific diets. Space considerations do not permit us to discuss all foods, and for this reason we tend to refer to food types, for example, leafy green vegetables, which includes a wide variety of choices. The diets outlined in Tables 8.2–8.4 will get you started thinking and eating right, and on the road toward total heart health. Having a consultation with an expert in the Maharishi Vedic Approach to Health will help refine and adapt some of these rules to your specific physiology and imbalances. (To locate a physician or practitioner in your area, see the Resources section.)

The specific diets recommended by the Vedic Approach are designed to balance your *predominant* imbalanced dosha. Pacifying the main aggravated dosha will help to correct the underlying imbalance that is likely to be contributing to your high blood pressure, high cholesterol, or other heart disease risk conditions. For example, if you have a Pitta imbalance, you have too much heat in your system and eating foods with heating properties, such as hot, spicy foods, will further increase the imbalance. The Pitta-pacifying diet includes foods that decrease Pitta, that is, that contain qualities that are opposite to Pitta. Eating foods with cooling properties, such as milk, wheat, and rice, will ease your current Pitta imbalance and help offset future imbalances.

How much of a dosha-pacifying food should you eat? The best gauge is to use your own experience. Ask yourself, "How do I feel?" If a particular food in a particular quantity in your diet makes you feel better, then that is probably right for you (unless it conflicts with a major guideline in this book). Note that the diets in the tables below suggest that you "include" or "favor" certain foods. Again, your experience (do you feel healthier and happier?) will help you refine these guidelines.

Some of the recommendations such as for spice mixtures give specific amounts and proportions with recipes. This is because concentrated spices can be more powerful than food alone, and you may need only small amounts of these. Also, diet alone without the spice mixtures may not be sufficient to correct severe dosha imbalances, but it will help and may be enough for mild imbalances. Where the imbalances are more severe, add several of the other methods such as spice mixtures, herbal preparations, and purification procedures presented later in Part Two to your daily routine and/or consider using all three approaches of the Total Heart Health program—the Mind, Body, and Environment Approaches. Also, for a complete diagnosis and set of personalized recommendations, a thorough evaluation by a Maharishi Vedic physician or practitioner is always recommended. Special formulations of medicinal plants may be used to supplement the diet with extra potent balancing effects on your physiology. These complex and highly refined mixtures of numerous herbal ingredients are used as nutritional supplements. In our clinical experience and review of the scientific literature, they are the best herbal supplements for correcting the basic imbalances that lead to heart disease and its risk factors. Ultimately, these herbal supplements work on the level of the inner intelligence of the body to re-enliven it in holistic and specific ways. (There's more about these special formulations in Chapter 9.)

However, whatever your current state of health and healthful interventions you are using, the Body Approach of the Total Heart Health program is complementary and prevention-oriented. The main point is that you adopt a diet and routine to pacify your predominant dosha. The Total Heart Health program includes three pacifying diets, each of which aims at balancing one of the doshas.

When following the dosha-specific diet for pacifying each dosha, you may want to review the qualities of that dosha and the tastes that pacify it. (Refer to pages 123–125.)

OPTIMIZING YOUR DIGESTION

The traditional texts of the Maharishi Vedic Approach to Health point out that the existence of heart disease and its risk factors usually indicates that ama has accumulated and ojas has decreased in the body. Ama, you may remember, is a sticky, toxic substance that results from poor digestion. Ojas, on the other hand, results from a balanced diet and strong digestion. It is a health-promoting substance that gives the body strength and resilience against disease. Once ama accumulates, it can travel throughout the body, blocking the channels or shrotas, such as the arteries in your heart. This blockage diminishes ojas, eventually causing coronary heart disease. Improving digestion, or agni, is instrumental in reducing ama. A robust digestive capacity can remove ama and eliminate impurities throughout the body.

Thus, the strength of your digestion is as important as the food you eat. A healthy and efficient digestive system enables you to fully metabolize and utilize the nutrients in the food. How you eat and when you eat have a great influence on this process. Here are some simple rules to follow to help ensure you get the maximum digestive power from your meals:

1. Eat your main meal at midday when your *agni,* or digestive fire, is strong-est. Eat lightly at night when digestion is not as strong. Eat meals at approximately the same time each day.

2. Prepare and cook meals in a settled environment, not in a chaotic, slap-dash manner.

3. Always sit to eat. Dine in a settled and quiet atmosphere. Do not work, read, drive, stand, or watch TV during meals.

4. Don't eat too quickly or too slowly.

5. Eat to about three-fourths of your capacity. Do not leave the table hungry or over full.

6. Avoid eating a meal until the previous meal is digested. Allow approxi-mately three to six hours between meals. Do not eat a meal unless you are hungry. An afternoon snack of fresh fruit, a few nuts, or other light, fresh food is all right.

7. Water, herbal teas, or fresh juices are fine to sip during meals.

8. Do not drink milk with a full meal, as it is best not to mix milk with most other tastes (especially salty and sour tastes). Milk may be consumed with sweet-tasting foods such as cereal and toast. Milk should never be con-sumed ice cold; it should always be heated (preferably boiled) before drink-ing to make it more digestible. For those with particular trouble digesting milk, you can add a pinch of cardamom, ginger, or turmeric, and dilute the milk with hot water.

9. Avoid ice-cold beverages or food. They interfere with digestion.

10. Avoid yogurt, cheese, cottage cheese, and buttermilk at night. These foods are heavy and difficult to digest. They are best eaten at the midday meal.

11. If you consume poultry or fish, eat these at lunch, around noon, when digestion is strongest and most efficient.

12. Do not eat heated or cooked honey. The heating process is said to cause a chemical reaction that leads to ama in the body.

13. Do not rush to leave the table after eating. Take a few minutes to sit qui-etly after finishing your meal.

TABLE 8.2. GUIDELINES FOR A VATA-PACIFYING DIET	
Food Types	Favor foods that are warm, heavy, and oily. Reduce foods that are cold, dry, and light.
Food Tastes	Include foods that are sweet, sour, and salty. Reduce foods that are spicy, bitter, and astringent.
Food Quantity	Eat larger quantities of food, but not more than you can digest easily.
Foods	**Animal protein:** No meat, including beef, pork, lamb, and veal. Poultry or fish if desired (in moderation) if digestion is strong.
	Beans and legumes: Reduce all beans in the diet, except for mung beans, preferably well cooked in the form of dahl, and tofu, a soybean byproduct.
	Dairy: All dairy products (whole milk is okay). Always boil milk before drinking to make it easier to digest; drink it warm. Do not consume milk with a complete meal.
	Fruits: Favor sweet, sour, or heavy fruits such as avocados, bananas, berries, cherries, grapes, mangoes, melons, oranges, papayas, peaches, pineapples, and plums. Reduce dry or light fruits such as apples, cranberries, pears, and pomegranates, including dried fruits.
	Grains: Rice and wheat are preferable. Reduce intake of barley, buckwheat, corn, millet, oats, and rye.
	Nuts and seeds: All nuts (in moderation).
	Oils: All oils in moderation. Ghee (clarified butter) and olive oil are especially recommended.
	Spices: Cardamom, cloves, cinnamon, cumin, ginger, mustard seed, salt, and small quantities of black pepper.
	Sweeteners: All natural sweeteners (in moderation), including honey, raw sugar, molasses, and others.
	Vegetables: Favor asparagus, beets, carrots, cucumbers, and sweet potatoes. Consume cooked, not raw. The following are acceptable in moderation if cooked with ghee or oil and Vata-pacifying spices: broccoli, cauliflower, celery, leafy green vegetables, peas, potatoes, and zucchini. Avoid cabbage and sprouts.

TABLE 8.3. GUIDELINES FOR A PITTA-PACIFYING DIET	
Food Types	Favor foods that are cooling and liquid. Reduce foods that are hot and spicy.
Food Tastes	Include foods that are sweet, bitter, or astringent. Reduce foods that create more heat, such as sour, spicy, and salty foods.
Food Quantity	Eat according to your appetite and as much as you can comfortably digest.
Foods	**Animal protein:** No meat, including beef, pork, lamb, and veal. Poultry or freshwater fish may be consumed if desired.
	Beans and legumes: Most common beans and legumes, except for miso, a fermented soybean product.
	Dairy: Milk, butter, and ghee. Reduce fermented foods with sour tastes such as buttermilk, cheese, sour cream, and yogurt.
	Fruits: Favor sweet fruits such as avocados, cherries, grapes, mangoes, melons, fully ripened oranges, pineapples, plums, and pomegranates. Reduce sour fruits such as grapefruits, olives, papayas, and unripe pineapples.
	Grains: Include barley, oats, wheat, and white rice in the diet. Reduce brown rice, corn, millet, and rye.
	Nuts and seeds: Almonds (blanched), coconut, flaxseeds, and sunflower seeds. Avoid all other nuts.
	Oils: Coconut, olive, and sunflower oils are best. Reduce use of almond, corn, and sesame oils.
	Spices and condiments: Cardamom, cinnamon, coriander, and fennel. Take black pepper, celery seed, clove, cumin, fenugreek, garlic, ginger, mustard seed, and salt only in small amounts. Avoid cayenne and chili peppers. Avoid ketchup, mayonnaise, mustard, pickles, and soy sauce.
	Sweeteners: All natural sweeteners (in moderation), except for honey and molasses.
	Vegetables: Include asparagus, broccoli, cauliflower, celery, cucumbers, green beans, leafy green vegetables, lettuce, okra, potatoes, pumpkins, sweet potatoes, and zucchini. Reduce beets, carrots, hot peppers, radishes, spinach, and tomatoes.

TABLE 8.4.   GUIDELINES FOR A KAPHA-PACIFYING DIET

Food Types	Favor foods that are light, dry, and warm. Reduce foods that are heavy, oily, and cold.
Food Tastes	Include foods that are spicy, bitter, and astringent. Reduce foods that are sweet, salty, and sour (for example, yogurt and cheese).
Food Quantity	Eat smaller quantities of food but enough to satisfy your hunger.
Foods	**Animal protein:** No meat, including beef, pork, lamb, and veal. Saltwater fish may be consumed in moderation if desired. Reduce poultry and freshwater fish.
	Beans and legumes: All beans and legumes, except tofu, a soybean byproduct.
	Dairy: Low-fat milk preferable. Always boil milk before drinking to make it easier to digest; drink warm. Do not drink milk with a complete meal or with sour or salty food tastes. If you use whole milk, add one or two pinches of turmeric or ginger and dilute in a 1:1 ratio with water before boiling to help reduce its kapha-increasing qualities.
	Fruits: Favor lighter fruits, such as apples and pears. Reduce heavy or sour fruits, such as avocados, bananas, coconuts, dates, figs, melons, oranges, and pineapples.
	Grains: Most grains, especially barley and millet. Reduce rice and wheat.
	Nuts and seeds: Reduce all nuts due to high oil content. Flaxseed, pumpkin seed, and sunflower seeds in moderation. Popcorn (without butter or salt).
	Oils: Almond, canola (organic only), corn, ghee, and sunflower oils are especially suitable.
	Spices: All spices, except salt.
	Sweeteners: Honey is best (use raw, not heated or cooked). Reduce all sugar products.
	Vegetables: All vegetables, except cucumbers, sweet potatoes, tomatoes, and zucchini.

WHAT TO EXPECT

Almost everyone will notice some positive effects soon after starting the proper dosha-balancing, heart-healthy diet. These might take the form of feeling lighter, happier, and more energetic in general. They are due to specific reductions in symptoms associated with the aggravated dosha that is now being pacified, which begins right away. Depending on the severity of the problem and how long it has persisted, people will experience symptomatic improvements after different times.

It is recommended that you stay on your dosha-pacifying diet long term. This is an eating plan that gives results cumulatively over time, not a short-term, quick-fix diet. It will reduce imbalances and prevent them from accumulating in the future. Staying on your dosha-pacifying diet should not be difficult because it is providing your body with what it needs and, as a result, should make you feel happy and healthy. Don't worry about occasionally going off your diet, such as when traveling. It may take a few weeks or even months to achieve your goal of a balanced physiology. You will feel better naturally and gradually as you wake up your body's inner intelligence.

CHAPTER 9 🝖

Specific Diets for Heart Disease and Its Risk Factors

SINCE, IN THE VIEW OF THE MAHARISHI VEDIC APPROACH to Health, heart disease and its risk factors are the results of dosha imbalances that have accumulated over a long time, the general dietary principles discussed in the previous chapter can be used either for preventing or reversing heart disease. In this chapter, we discuss how the Total Heart Health diet may be tailored specifically to your health condition, that is, to your particular risk-factor profile or heart disease state. This includes using highly targeted diets as well as specific teas, spices, and herbal supplements, all of which contain different and complementary packets of nature's intelligence. Once again, the key principle is to enliven the body's inner intelligence. Ideally, these guidelines for diet and supplements are to be integrated into your Total Heart Health program, which includes the Mind, Body, and Environment Approaches.

Having established the general dietary principles for creating health and avoiding imbalance and disease, we're now ready to show you how to modify these principles for treating or preventing heart disease and its risk factors. Those with heart disease will want to reduce the dosha imbalances causing their disease (see Table 9.1). Those with risk factors will want to reduce the imbalances causing their risk factors (see Tables 9.2–9.6), which will, in turn, prevent heart disease. Remember to consult with your doctor about how these the Maharishi Vedic Approach to Health recommendations fit in with your conventional medical care.

The guidelines presented in this chapter are designed to supplement the core Vata-, Pitta-, and Kapha-pacifying diets described in the previous chapter. If you have more than one risk factor, or heart disease plus one or more risk factors, then follow the appropriate dosha-pacifying diet for your major imbalance,

but you may also add other specific recommendations such as herbal supplements from the heart disease or risk-factor categories. Likewise, if you have
more than one dosha that is out of balance, the recommended approach is to
start using the core diet designed to pacify the dosha you identified in Chapter
7 as being the most aggravated in your physiology. After a few months, you
may recheck what your predominant dosha imbalance is by filling out the questionnaires on pages 109–111 once again. More intensive programs may be recommended and supervised by a Maharishi Vedic physician or practitioner (see
the Resources section).

The guidelines presented in the following tables focus on special foods, teas,
spice mixtures (also called *churnas*), and herbs and herbal supplements that
are highly useful in balancing specific dosha imbalances. Sources and additional
information for the herbal preparations, dosha-specific teas and churnas, and
aromatic oils mentioned in the tables are available from Maharishi Ayurveda
Products International (MAPI, see the Resources section). Recommendations for
certain dishes and spice mixtures followed by an asterisk (*) are presented in the
next chapter. Recommendations for lifestyle and daily and seasonal routines that
will help ameliorate dosha disorders and restore balance to your heart health will
be presented in Chapter 11. Unless otherwise noted, use the following general
guidelines for teas, spice mixtures, and herbal preparations:

- For teas: Consume 1 to 3 cups daily.

- For spice mixtures: 1 teaspoon per serving.

- For herbal supplements: The dose schedule is usually 1 to 2 tablets (or 1 to
  2 teaspoons) twice daily. But always read the label or follow the specific
  advice of an expert in the Maharishi Vedic Approach to Health.

RECOMMENDATIONS FOR TARGETING HEART DISEASE

The following guidelines are for those who presently have heart disease. By
"heart disease," we mean atherosclerosis (blockage of the arteries) that has led
to coronary heart disease. This includes those who have had a heart attack,
bypass surgery, angioplasty, and/or positive results on angiography, stress tests,
or other tests for heart disease.

While modern medicine studies and treats the physical heart, the Maharishi
Vedic Approach to Health recognizes and addresses two aspects of the heart:
the physical organ that pumps blood throughout the body and the emotional
organ that experiences happiness, love, and sorrow. Even more deeply, the
traditional texts of Vedic physiology indicate that the heart is the seat of ojas,
that subtle, life-sustaining substance we described earlier. Ojas provides basic
strength, immunity, defense against disease, and emotional bliss or happiness.

Each of the doshas is involved in the heart's structure and function. An imbalance in any of the three doshas can result in heart disease. For example, Vata, the principle of movement, governs the rhythmic beating of the heart and circulation of blood in the arteries throughout the body. Pitta governs the emotions and their influences on heart functioning. Kapha is responsible for the structure, stability, and muscular strength of the heart.

When Vata dosha becomes aggravated by the fast pace of modern life, mental stress, irregular routine, or other factors, it may cause narrowing of the arteries through spasm, also called *vasoconstriction* in modern medicine. A person may experience this as a tightening or gripping type of chest pain. This type of angina may also be provoked by mental stress.

If an individual is experiencing chronic emotional stress, or indulging in a Pitta-aggravating diet or lifestyle, then Pitta dosha in the heart may become imbalanced. This causes a cascade of metabolic and enzymatic reactions resulting in the buildup of Pitta-related toxins, or ama, in the arteries. This ancient description may correspond to the modern concept of inflammation, which is now believed to play a major role in atherosclerosis. People with Pitta-type heart disease may experience a burning type of discomfort or pain during an episode of angina. Indeed, some people classically experience their angina as "heartburn." Pitta-type heart disease may also be experienced as sharp chest pain during physical exertion or emotional stress.

Kapha-type heart disease may be due to overindulgence in unhealthy fatty foods. This results in higher levels of ama, which clogs the arteries. In modern terminology, this would correspond to cholesterol in the blood and cholesterol deposits in the plaques that cause obstruction to the blood flow in the coronary arteries.

Most serious heart disease in contemporary society is thought to be caused by mental or emotional stress (Vata or Pitta aggravations). In addition, a diet that is high in fats or in the wrong type of fats may cause a Kapha imbalance by itself or in combination with one or two of the other dosha imbalances.

Since heart disease can be due to imbalances in any of the three doshas in different people, as we described in Chapter 7, Table 9.1 (and all subsequent tables in this chapter) gives recommendations according to your predominant dosha imbalance.

To reduce or reverse the major risk factors associated with heart disease (hypertension, high cholesterol, stress, obesity, diabetes, menopause), start by following one of the dosha-pacifying diets (Tables 8.2–8.4) according to your results from the questionnaires in Chapter 7. Then, follow the additional guidelines listed in the appropriate tables in this chapter. These tables contain new information and emphasize earlier recommendations.

TABLE 9.1. SPECIFIC RECOMMENDATIONS FOR HEART DISEASE

Additional Guidelines for a Vata-Pacifying Diet

Foods	*Follow the guidelines for a Vata-pacifying diet in Table 8.2, page 123, with the following modifications:*
Increase	Freshly cooked, warm, moist, not dry foods; sweet fruits, especially pears and mangoes; nuts, especially soaked walnuts and almonds; grains, especially amaranth and barley; vegetables, especially asparagus, artichokes, broccoli, and zucchini.
Decrease	No additional guidelines.
Other	Eat home-cooked meals.
Herbs and Oils	Take *Cardio Support* tablets; *Worry Free* tablets; and *Blissful Sleep I* tablets at bedtime, if experiencing insomnia; take *Maharishi Amrit Kalash®*; use *Worry Free* aroma oil.
Spices	Season food with *Vata Churna* or Vata-Pacifying Spice Mixture*.
Teas	Drink *Vata Tea*.

Additional Guidelines for a Pitta-Pacifying Diet

Foods	*Follow the guidelines for a Pitta-pacifying diet in Table 8.3, page 124, with the following modifications:*
Increase	Stewed pears* for breakfast; sweet, juicy pears as snacks; *Rose Petal Preserve;* sweet lassi* or date milk shakes*; ripe mangoes; summer squash.
Decrease	Spicy, sour, salty foods; winter squashes; large-sized legumes such as kidney beans, dried yellow and green peas; tofu; ketchup, mustard, salad dressings, and other foods made with vinegar.
Other	Avoid delaying or skipping meals; drink lots of pure water throughout the day; eat fresh foods.
Herbs and Oils	Take *Cardio Support* tablets; *Blissful Joy* (1 tablet if taking with *Cardio Support*); use *Blissful Joy* aroma oil; take *Blissful Sleep 2* tablets at bedtime, if unable to sleep; take *Maharishi Amrit Kalash*.
Spices	Season food with either *Pitta Churna* or Pitta-Pacifying Spice Mixture*.
Teas	Drink *Pitta Tea*.

Additional Guidelines for a Kapha-Pacifying Diet

Foods	*Follow the guidelines for a Kapha-pacifying diet in Table 8.4, page 125, with the following modifications:*
Increase	Astringent, pungent tastes; stewed apples* or pears* for breakfast; grains, especially amaranth; cooked leafy green vegetables such as chard, spinach, and kale.

Decrease	Sweet, sour, and salty foods; all cold foods and drinks; heavy desserts (eat fruit instead).
Other	Eat fresh, warm, well-cooked, easily digestible foods with small amounts of ghee* or olive oil.
Herbs and Oils	Take *Elim-Tox O* tablets; use *Blissful Sleep 3* tablets at bedtime; take *Maharishi Amrit Kalash;* use *Fatigue Free* aroma oil.
Spices	Season food with ghee* and either *Kapha Churna* or Kapha-Pacifying Spice Mixture*.
Teas	Drink *Kapha Tea.*

Additional Guidelines for All Dosha Imbalances

Fats	Reduce fats, especially animal fat, and increase your consumption of vegetables. If you do this and favor fresh, whole, organic foods, you will largely eliminate "bad" or unhealthy fats. These include saturated fats, partially hydrogenated "trans" fats (found in margarines and packaged foods and commercial baked goods), and foods high in cholesterol (for example, red meat and butter), which raise blood levels of "bad" cholesterol (LDL). Avoid rancid and overheated fats, which produce large numbers of free radicals.
Protein	If you are following a vegetarian diet that includes no meat, chicken, fish, or eggs, be sure to get adequate protein. This is easily achieved because many widely available foods contain significant amounts of protein. Substantial amounts of protein can be found in dairy products such as lassi*, milk, and cheese (especially favor panir*, a type of fresh cheese that can be made at home from cow's milk; ricotta; or other nonaged cheeses), legumes (beans, peas, or lentils), tofu (soy cheese), grains (wheat germ, rice, barley, quinoa, breads, pasta), and all nuts and seeds. Eating a variety of these foods will provide you with all of the essential amino acids, which are the building blocks of protein.
Heart-Nourishing Foods	Emphasize foods that are especially nourishing to the heart: mature, fresh pomegranate fruit or juice; asparagus; sweet, juicy, seasonal fruits; *Rose Petal Preserve;* sweet lassi*; avocadoes; and leafy green vegetables
Spice Mixtures	When cooking vegetables, season with the *Healthy Heart Spice Mixture** or recommended dosha-specific spice mixtures*.

* See Chapter 10 for recipe.

RECOMMENDATIONS FOR LOWERING HIGH BLOOD PRESSURE

According to the ancient Vedic approach to health, hypertension is one sign of disorder in the cardiovascular system, but the underlying causes may be different in different people, depending on which doshas are out of balance. For some, the cause of their hypertension will be a Vata imbalance that is worsened by a Vata-aggravating diet and lifestyle. Taxing the mind with too much mental work or too much mental stress aggravates Vata. Other contributing factors might include not getting enough sleep, working late or watching TV late at night, constantly dividing the mind by doing two things at once (such as talking on the phone while cooking or driving), rushing from one thing to the next, feeling the pressure of too little time, and exercising too much for your body type. Contributing dietary causes might include eating too many dry, light, or raw foods; skipping too many meals; having no set mealtime; eating while standing up, while doing business, or while talking on the phone; and, in general, not eating enough.

Similarly, there are Pitta-related causes for high blood pressure. An excess of Pitta can cause more reactive, aggravated changes in the heart and blood vessels. Sometimes Pitta aggravation is related to food-derived toxins that accumulate in the liver. When Pitta is aggravated, people have less capacity to cope with emotional challenges, and their blood pressure goes up. Some lifestyle habits that might cause this to happen are going to bed late, watching disturbing movies, and too much emotional stress. As for diet, eating too many spicy, hot foods such as chilis and jalapeno peppers can aggravate Pitta dosha. You should also avoid too much sour food such as ketchup, mustard, vinegar-based salad dressings, sour oranges, grapes, or lemons, and highly salty foods such as chips, cheeses, and most processed foods. In general, foods that are not "intelligent" such as processed foods and nonorganic foods grown with chemicals and pesticides overtax the liver and cause Pitta to go out of balance.

Of course, there are also Kapha-related causes for high blood pressure. If digestion is weak and ama, a waste product of incomplete digestion, has been present in the body for a long time, it can spread to the fat tissue and mix with Kapha in the heart region. This kind of ama-induced imbalance blocks the shrotas, the channels that circulate oxygen throughout the body and also causes high blood pressure. In this situation, it is extremely important to examine your diet and switch to healthier fats, such as ghee and olive oil in moderation. It is the unhealthy fats, the fats found in red meat and the trans fats such as hydrogenated vegetable oil found in almost all packaged foods, which cause this kind of ama/Kapha imbalance. Also, you should switch from using refined sugar and packaged sweets to using healthier sweeteners. Honey pacifies Kapha (but do not cook with honey because this releases toxins into an otherwise pure and light food). Other foods to avoid are hard cheeses and whole milk and butter. For a person with a Kapha imbalance, it is important to exercise every day (see Chapter 12 for Kapha-specific exercises). Try to keep some variety in your diet. Follow the dietary recommendations to pacify Kapha dosha to open the channels. It is essential that the arteries be clear of ama (the toxic byproduct of improper digestion) and blockage, because even if a Kapha-predominant person has more ojas (the nourishing byproduct of proper digestion), it cannot reach the targeted areas of the heart to give it support as and when needed if the channels are blocked.

Table 9.2 gives the dietary choices to avoid and to favor for each type of imbalance causing hypertension. Gentle lifestyle changes that are recommended are discussed in Chapter 11. People who have a certain dosha imbalance will need to be more careful to avoid the things that aggravate that particular imbalance.

RECOMMENDATIONS FOR REDUCING HIGH CHOLESTEROL

From the viewpoint of the Maharishi Vedic Approach to Health, high cholesterol is primarily due to an excess of Kapha. However, in certain individuals, Vata or Pitta dosha may also be aggravated. If this is the case, it's recommended that you follow the Vata- or Pitta-pacifying diets described in the previous chapter in Tables 8.2 and 8.3, respectively. After your Vata or Pitta dosha becomes balanced, then follow a Kapha-pacifying diet, in addition to following the cholesterol-lowering dietary recommendations below and in Table 9.3. In other words, follow the Vata-pacifying or Pitta-pacifying diet first if the questionnaires on pages 109–111 show that you have a predominance of aggravated Vata or Pitta. If, of course, they show a predominance of aggravated Kapha, then start with the Kapha-pacifying program in Table 8.4 and follow the additional recommendations in Table 9.3 for targeting high cholesterol for those with a Kapha imbalance.

Some of the more important dietary recommendations previously discussed for lowering cholesterol include eating your meals at the same time every day and having your largest meal at lunchtime when your digestion is strong. To avoid indigestion at night, eat lightly in the evenings. Additional dietary recommendations are discussed below.

Consume a yogurt drink called *lassi* daily. While this may seem to conflict with some of our previous recommendations to avoid yogurt, lassi is actually helpful for lowering cholesterol. Although yogurt is difficult to digest and clogs the channels (due to its heaviness and sourness), blending yogurt with water and spices to make lassi actually changes its properties, making the yogurt lighter, easier to digest, and pacifying for all of the doshas. A recipe for making

TABLE 9.2. SPECIFIC RECOMMENDATIONS FOR HYPERTENSION

Additional Guidelines for a Vata-Pacifying Diet

Foods	*Follow the additional dietary guidelines for a Vata-pacifying diet with specific recommendations for heart disease in Table 9.1, page 130, with the following modifications:*
Increase	Heavier, fuller meals, and moderate amounts of unctuous, sweet, salty, and sour foods.
Decrease	Spicy, pungent foods.
Other	Establish a regular daily routine especially for mealtimes and bedtime.
Herbs and Oils	In addition to the herbs, teas, and supplements recommended in Table 9.1, take *BP Balance* tablets; use *Herbal Cleanse* tablets if constipated and *Herbal Aci-Balance* tablets if bloated or constipated.

Additional Guidelines for a Pitta-Pacifying Diet

Foods	*Follow the additional dietary guidelines for a Pitta-pacifying diet with specific recommendations for heart disease in Table 9.1, page 130, with the following modifications:*
Increase	Sweet and juicy fruits; cooling vegetables such as asparagus, zucchini, yellow squash, loki squash, and broccoli. In the hot season, cool your mind and emotions with sweet and juicy fruits, such as watermelon, and drink lots of water.
Decrease	Avoid spicy and sour foods.
Other	Establish a regular daily routine especially for mealtimes and bedtime.
Herbs and Oils	In addition to the herbs, teas, and supplements recommended in Table 9.1, take *BP Balance* tablets and use *Herbal Aci-Balance* tablets if experiencing heartburn.

Additional Guidelines For A Kapha-Pacifying Diet

Foods	*Follow the additional dietary guidelines for a Kapha-pacifying diet with specific recommendations for heart disease in Table 9.1, page 130, with the following modifications:*
Increase	Use only healthy fats such as ghee* and olive oil in moderation. Use honey as a sweetener (but not for cooking).
Decrease	Avoid all harmful fats such as in red meat and hydrogenated oils. Avoid all packaged, processed, and frozen foods. Avoid refined sugars. Avoid hard cheeses and butter. Whole milk may be diluted 1:1 with water for a low-fat drink. Boil then cool before drinking.
Other	Go for variety in your diet and routine.
Herbs, Oils, Spices, and Teas	No additional guidelines.

digestive lassi is given in Chapter 10 on page 156. Drink this after lunch, and it will help bolster the healthy microbes that aid digestion. This is especially important if you are taking *Cholesterol Protection* tablets and detoxifying the liver, because the toxins will be eliminated through the colon. Digestive lassi will help to clear out the toxins more quickly.

Be sure to use the Cholesterol-Lowering Spice Mixture in preparing your main dish or side dishes (see Chapter 10 for recipe). Combine the spice mixture with vegetables or grains to give them a satisfying flavor and enhance digestion. Add salt to taste.

For breakfast, have a cooked or stewed apple, to which you can add cooked prunes and figs that help to cleanse the bowel and eliminate cholesterol. Use ghee and/or olive oil for cooking in general.

RECOMMENDATIONS FOR RELIEVING STRESS

In the Total Heart Health program, we target the causal factors to bring the system back into balance. Stress can be of three types: mental, emotional, and physical. Each requires different treatment approaches. Vata governs the mind, so mental stress aggravates Vata dosha mostly. Pitta governs the emotions, so emotional stress aggravates Pitta dosha primarily. Kapha governs the structure of the body, so physical stress has its effects primarily on Kapha dosha.

Mental stress is traditionally thought to be caused by an overuse or misuse of the mind. For instance, if you perform intense mental work many hours a day or if you work long hours on a computer, it can cause an imbalance in Vata, the physiological operator concerned with brain activity. The first symptom of Vata imbalance is a reduced ability to handle stressful situations. As the person feels more and more distressed, his or her mental functions such as acquisition, retention, and recall are diminished. The person's mind becomes hyperactive, yet the person loses the ability to remember, to make clear decisions, to think positively, to feel enthusiastic, and even to fall asleep at night. To treat mental stress, you should begin by managing your behavior and your mental activity that cause this dosha to become aggravated (for suggestions see Behaviors for Heart Health on page 179 in Chapter 11). Second, you can take measures presented in Table 9.4 to pacify Vata-type stress.

Emotional stress can be caused by a problem in a relationship, the loss of a friend or relative, or any situation that might hurt your feelings. Emotional stress shows up as irritability, depression, and emotional instability. It affects sleep in a different way than mental stress; it can cause you to wake up in the middle of the night and not be able to go back to sleep. With emotional stress, the management is quite different. Emotional stress disturbs Pitta, the physiological operator concerned with the emotions and functioning of the heart. To balance

TABLE 9. 3. SPECIFIC RECOMMENDATIONS FOR HIGH CHOLESTEROL

Additional Guidelines for a Vata-Pacifying Diet

Foods	Follow a Vata-pacifying diet (Table 8.2, page 123), but only until Vata is balanced and/or in Vata season (November–February, for information on seasonal routines, see Chapter 11). Then switch to a Kapha-pacifying diet (Table 8.4, page 125) and follow the cholesterol-lowering dietary guidelines for all dosha types below (see last section in table).
Increase	At breakfast, eat a stewed apple* to cleanse the bowel and to lower cholesterol.
Decrease	Oils and fats (even though they are Vata pacifying)
Herbs, Oils, Spices, and Teas	Use Vata spice and tea; after Vata is balanced, use the Cholesterol-Lowering Spice Mixture*; take *Maharishi Amrit Kalash.*

Additional Guidelines for a Pitta-Pacifying Diet

Foods	Follow a Pitta-pacifying diet (Table 8.3, page 124) until Pitta is balanced. Then switch to a Kapha-pacifying diet (Table 8.4, page 125) and incorporate the cholesterol-lowering suggestions below. At breakfast, eat a stewed apple* to cleanse the bowel and lower cholesterol.
Decrease	Oils and fats
Herbs, Oils, Spices, and Teas	Take *Maharishi Amrit Kalash,* and use Pitta spices and tea. After Pitta is balanced, use the Cholesterol-Lowering Spice Mixture.*

Additional Guidelines for a Kapha-Pacifying Diet

Foods	*Follow the Kapha-pacifying diet in Table 8.4, page 125 with the following modifications:*
Increase	Favor light, dry, and warm foods. At breakfast, eat a stewed apple* to cleanse the bowel and lower cholesterol.
Decrease	Reduce heavy, oily, cold foods and sweet, sour and salty tastes.
Herb, Oils, Spices, and Teas	Use Cholesterol-Lowering Spice Mixture* and *Kapha Tea.*

Additional Guidelines for All Dosha Imbalances

Foods	Drink warm water throughout the day. Drink digestive lassi* every day (for example, with lunch or afternoon snack). Eat cooked food, and eat it warm. Avoid saturated fats, trans fats, and high-cholesterol foods. Avoid rancid and overheated fats. Cook with small amounts of ghee* or olive oil. Milk recommendations: Boil milk (preferably organic) with an equal amount of water and pinches of ground cardamom and cinnamon for five minutes. Sip slowly when warm, but cool enough

	to drink. If you crave sweets, eat sweet and juicy fruits. Do not skip meals as this can aggravate the liver where cholesterol is processed.
Herbs, Oils, Spices, and Teas	Take *Cholesterol Protection* tablets. Take psyllium husk (1–2 tablespoons in water before bed) or high-fiber wheat or oat bran with cereals or vegetables daily; take *Maharishi Amrit Kalash*.

* See Chapter 10 for recipe.

emotional stress, you need to favor Pitta-pacifying foods and routines. Dietary recommendations are given in Table 9.4. Lifestyle recommendations are provided in Chapter 11.

Physical stress is caused by the misuse or overuse of the body, such as exercising too much or working for extended periods at a job that is physically taxing. A person experiencing physical fatigue may also experience mental fogginess, difficulty in concentrating, and dullness of the mind. Excessive physical strain causes both Kapha and Vata dosha types to go out of balance. Kapha is concerned with lubrication of the joints, the muscular system, and moisture balance in the skin. Vata governs circulation and the nervous system. Another cause of physical stress is too little exercise, which results in a sluggish digestion and the formation of ama, the digestive impurities that clog the channels. In either case, the process of regenerating cells slows down, and thus the cells themselves become physically tired. The solution is to balance both Kapha and Vata to stabilize and nourish the body.

RECOMMENDATIONS FOR LOSING EXCESS WEIGHT

Being overweight or obese can be due to a Vata, Pitta, or Kapha imbalance. The Total Heart Health program does not focus on appetite suppression or calorie reduction typical of most weight-loss programs. It does not target suppressing the appetite because doing that slows down fat metabolism. If the body does not assimilate fat and carbohydrates effectively, then fat and impurities accumulate in the body as excess weight. It does not target calorie reduction because that typically leads to the "yo-yo effect," a term used to describe the phenomenon in which individuals, who, after dieting, return to their previous eating patterns (which almost all of them do) and gain back the weight they lost and more! And the underlying imbalances are still there.

Instead, our recommendations focus on correcting the primary dosha imbalance that is causing the problem. In kind, the Total Heart Health approach to weight management not only helps you achieve a healthy weight, but it also results in side benefits such as increased stamina, a more efficiently functioning body, and youthful appearance. It is suggested that people who want to bal-

TABLE 9.4. SPECIFIC RECOMMENDATIONS FOR STRESS

Additional Guidelines for Mental Stress

Foods	*Follow the Vata-pacifying diet in Table 8.2, page 123, with the following modifications:*
Increase	Start the day with a stewed apple* to cleanse the bowel. Eat foods that pacify Vata and specifically strengthen the brain, including: ghee* and olive oil, milk, coconut milk, sweet summer squashes, fresh juicy seasonal fruits, soaked almonds and sunflower seeds, walnuts, raisins and dates, date milk shakes*, mango milk shakes (see variation of date milk shake), and rice pudding.
Decrease	Avoid caffeine, alcohol, and tobacco. Avoid unintelligent foods such as junk food, canned and packaged foods, and leftovers.
Other	Eat two to three warm, nourishing meals a day at regular times. Drink lots of warm liquids. Avoid cold, iced, and carbonated drinks.
Herbs and Oils	Take *Worry Free* tablets; use *Mind Power* liquid or *Mind Flex* tablets. Drink lots of warm water. Drink Herbal Brain Water*, which helps deliver nutrients to the deep tissues of the brain, and sip it throughout the day. Take *Maharishi Amrit Kalash*.
Spices	Use *Vata Churna* with meals, and Mental Stress-Relief Spice Mixture* to enhance the absorption and assimilation of nutrients and support the brain.
Teas	Drink *Worry Free Tea*. Use *Vata Tea;* it is calming.

Additional Guidelines for Emotional Stress

Foods	*Follow the Pitta-pacifying diet in Table 8.3, page 124, with the following modifications:*
Increase	Start the day with a stewed apple*. Use ghee* regularly. Eat lots of sweet and juicy fruits.
Decrease	Avoid junk or unintelligent foods, such as leftovers and canned, frozen, or packaged foods. People with emotional stress might be particularly prone to consuming these foods.
Other	Drink plenty of water.
Herb and Oils	Take *Herbal Cleanse* tablets at night. Try sweet lassi* with *Rose Petal Preserve* at the noon meal; drink a cup of warm milk with *Rose Petal Preserve* before bed. Take the *Blissful Joy* herbal tablets. Use *Maharishi Amrit Kalash*.
Spices	Use the Emotional Stress-Relief Spice Mixture*.

Additional Guidelines for Physical Stress

Foods	*Follow the Kapha-pacifying diet in Table 8.4, page 125, but take some Vata-pacifying foods (sweet, sour, salty taste) in moderation.*

Increase	Certain foods are also natural stress busters. These include walnuts, almonds, coconut, any sweet and juicy seasonal fruit such as pears and apples (stewed if possible); milk, lassi*, ghee*, and fresh cheeses, such as panir or ricotta.
Decrease	No additional guidelines.
Herbs and Oils	Take *Stress Free Body* and *Worry Free* herbal tablets. Take the *Deep Rest* herbal tablets to help wake up refreshed.
Teas	Sip *Vata* or *Kapha Tea* throughout the day. *Take Maharishi Amrit Kalash.*

See Chapter 10 for recipe.

ance their weight first identify which "type" of weight gain below best describes them, and then follow the corresponding guidelines in Table 9.5.

- **Kapha-type weight gain:** The first type of overweight imbalance is due to a lack of digestive fire (low agni) and low metabolic activity. These individuals, even though they may eat very small amounts of food, tend to gain weight. Two things are happening: (1) digestive impurities are being created, and (2) fat tissue is accumulating in the body. This is a very common weight problem, and the solution is to follow an ama-burning, toxin-eliminating program as outlined in the Kapha-pacifying diet.

- **Pitta-type weight gain:** The second type of overweight imbalance occurs when a person has long-term ama buildup and the channels around the stomach have been clogged, creating too much heat in the body. Here, the appetite may be very high and the individual may experience a lot of thirst. The person may also experience heartburn or other Pitta-aggravated imbalances, such as irritability and impatience. These individuals should be on a Pitta-pacifying diet. Herbal water (see Chapter 10 for recipe) assists the thermogenic (fat-burning) process, fenugreek burns fat and helps absorption, coriander eliminates toxins, and licorice is cooling and fennel helps with digestion.

- **Vata-type weight gain:** If you are Vata predominant, you are normally thin and wiry. But that does not mean weight gain will never be a problem for you. Sometimes Vata types are thin all their lives and then suddenly put on weight because their metabolism has changed. Vata-predominant people are susceptible to mental stress because they tend to overuse or misuse their minds. When under stress, they also tend to forget to eat regularly, thus disturbing their digestion, creating ama, and clogging the channels. This is often the precursor to weight gain. These people should follow the Vata-pacifying diet.

TABLE 9.5. SPECIFIC RECOMMENDATIONS FOR OBESITY

Additional Guidelines for a Vata-Pacifying Diet

Foods	*Follow the Vata-pacifying diet described in Table 8.2, page 123, with the following modifications:*
Increase	Eat foods that are fresh, organic, and whole. For breakfast, try stewed apples* and/or stewed pears*. For dinner, eat whole grains and soups made with fresh vegetables and pulses. For the main meal at noon, include organic vegetables such as zucchini and loki squash, grains such as quinoa, light proteins such as split mung dahl side dish* or soup*, and light dairy products such as lassi* and panir.
Decrease	Avoid foods that are too heavy (aged cheeses, meats, and heavy desserts). Avoid foods that are too light and dry (crackers, cold cereals, and packaged snacks).
Other	Nourish the body with light, easily digestible food. Take three warm, cooked meals a day, at the same time every day.
Herb and Oils	Use *Be Trim 3* tablets. Drink herbal water* throughout the day. Use *Vital Woman* or *Vital Man* tablets, and *Worry Free* tablets. Cook with light, nourishing oils such as ghee and olive oil.
Spices	Cook with turmeric, coriander, cumin, and fennel.
Teas	Drink *Be Trim* and *Worry Free Teas.*

Additional Guidelines for a Pitta-Pacifying Diet

Foods	*Follow the Pitta-pacifying diet described in Table 8.3, page 124, with the following modifications:*
Increase	Include sweet and juicy fruits, squash, warm milk, and homemade buttermilk* in the diet. Eat stewed prunes and figs (prepared similar to recipe for stewed apples) on weekends for gentle laxative therapy.
Decrease	No additional guidelines.
Herb and Oils	Use *Be Trim 2* supplements. Drink herbal water. Prepare as described above.
Spices	When cooking vegetables, use heart-healthy spice mixture* or *Pitta Churna* or Pitta-Pacifying Spice Mixture.*
Teas	Drink *Be Trim Tea.*

Additional Guidelines for a Kapha-Pacifying Diet

Foods	*Follow the Kapha-pacifying diet in Table 8.4 on page 125 with the following modifications:*
Herbs and Oils	Use *Be Trim 1* tablets. Weekly, use a gentle laxative therapy such as *Herbal Cleanse* tablets.

Spices	Cook with heart-healthy spice mixture* or *Kapha Churna* or Kapha Spice Mixture*.
Teas	Drink *Be Trim Tea.*

Additional Guidelines for All Dosha Imbalances	
Foods	Limit fat to 2 teaspoons of ghee* or olive oil per day (1 teaspoon at lunch, 1 teaspoon at dinner). For lunch and dinner, make 50 percent of your meal vegetables; 20 percent power grains (quinoa, whole barley, oats, millet, amaranth); and 30 percent high-protein foods such as lentils, panir, or nuts. Eat until nearly full. Add barley soup and mung bean dahl soup* to your diet. Eat sweet and juicy fruits daily as recommended for a Vata, Pitta, or Kapha diet.
Increase	Take two cups of hot or warm milk per day (may dilute milk 1:1 with water). Take a small cup of lassi* at lunch to balance Pitta. Emotional stress will be reduced. Drink barley water or kanji water* during the day to cleanse the system, for energy, and to help with hunger. Eat live protein filled with intelligence of nature from almonds (no more than ten per day), walnuts, legumes, sunflower seeds, sesame seeds, pumpkin seeds, and dairy products. Almond butter and *Almond Energy Drink* are delicious ways to boost your energy.
Decrease	Avoid commercial protein-powder drinks. Reduce or avoid meat. Avoid cold beverages, aged cheese, potatoes, yeasted breads, butter, cookies, cakes, ice cream, chocolates, deep-fried food, and cream sauces. Reduce intake of rice. Avoid leftovers and frozen, canned, packaged, and processed foods.
Other	Have patience. Once the digestive fire is strong and your metabolic processes are balanced, you can be more flexible with your diet.
Herbs, Oils, Spices, and Teas	To avoid overeating due to emotional stress, take *Blissful Joy* tablets to uplift the emotions or *Worry Free* tablets and tea to avoid overeating due to anxious thoughts. For sugar cravings, try 1 teaspoon *Rose Petal Preserve*, *Be Trim Tea*, one date, or a small amount of lassi*. Cook with fennel, cumin, coriander, and turmeric. Instead of coffee or tea, try an antioxidant coffee substitute such as *Rajas Cup* or a dosha-specific herbal tea.

See Chapter 10 for recipe.

Common to both Vata and Pitta types of weight gain is overeating due to stress, either mental or emotional. This can manifest as eating when you are not hungry or looking for something sweet to pacify a bad mood. If this is the case, follow the respective guidelines for mental and emotional stress in Table 9.4 and the specific recommendations for obesity in Table 9.5. *Blissful Joy* tablets will help to uplift your emotions; *Worry Free* tablets and *Worry Free Tea* will help you avoid overeating due to anxious thoughts. A teaspoon of *Rose Petal*

Preserve, Be Trim Tea, one date, or a little lassi will also help if you experience sugar cravings. Avoid commercial protein-powder drinks. Instead, eat live protein filled with the intelligence of nature from almonds (no more than ten per day), walnuts, legumes, sunflower seeds, sesame seeds, pumpkin seeds, and dairy products.

These guidelines get to the root of the problem by balancing fat and carbohydrate metabolism to help your body break down your stores of fat. Following these guidelines will slow down the digestion of carbohydrates, so you won't crave sweets and overeat, and you'll have more energy. You'll maintain a good appetite and absorb the nutrients you need to stay healthy and balanced. Patience is also one of the key factors that should be included in this program. This is not a fast method to shed pounds, but a holistic, natural approach from which you will see satisfying results gradually. Once the digestive fire is strong and the metabolic processes are balanced, then you may enjoy a little more leniency with your diet.

RECOMMENDATIONS FOR MENOPAUSE

After menopause, coronary heart disease increases dramatically among women. For this reason, menopause may be considered a risk factor for heart disease. Menopause is a gradual process that occurs over a period of time as a woman's ovaries stop producing estrogen. During this time, it's important to prevent or reduce any accumulation of ama to avoid the short- and long-term effects of a hormone imbalance, such as a blockage of the coronary arteries in the heart. The Vata-pacifying dietary recommendations and the rejuvenation treatments discussed in detail in Chapter 12 are especially effective in balancing the transformation of the dhatus, or tissues, at the onset of menopause. With this, effects of imbalanced tissues, such as heart disease, may be prevented.

Although each individual has a genetic predisposition toward a particular dosha predominance, there are many factors that can increase or decrease the doshas. We have already seen how food, behavior, and stress can be such factors. Age is another.

The Maharishi Vedic Approach to Health maintains that there are three stages of life for both men and women. In the first trimester of life—youth—the body's structure is developed to maturity and Kapha dosha, the dosha concerned with structure, tends to be increased. In the second stage—adulthood—most people achieve their peak in terms of productivity and creativity, and, not surprisingly, Pitta dosha tends to be increased. The third trimester of life is synonymous with the senior years, and Vata dosha tends to be increased. Menopause takes place during the transition between the Pitta stage and the Vata stage of life; that is, between middle age and the third trimester of life.

Because menopause typically occurs toward the end of the Pitta stage and the beginning of Vata stage, it is common for a menopausal woman to experience both Vata- and Pitta-related imbalances. For instance, menopausal complaints such as insomnia, memory lapses, anxiety, vaginal dryness, and aging skin are all related to an imbalance in Vata dosha. Pitta-related imbalances are experienced in menopause as hot flashes, urinary tract infections, anger, irritability, hyperacidity, and skin breakouts and rashes. If a woman already has a significant Pitta or Vata imbalance in the years before menopause, her symptoms are likely to be much, much worse.

Another factor leading to menopausal imbalances is the accumulation of ama in the body, typically caused by improper diet. Ama contributes to disease and aging, including menopausal problems. If a woman has had problems in the years before menopause with an accumulation of ama, then her symptoms of menopause are likely to be worse. A third factor is the misuse or overuse of the mind, body, emotions, or senses. This happens when a woman strains her mind too much (mental stress), is under too much ongoing stress or pressure (emotional stress), or is doing work that is too physically demanding (physical stress). These preexisting imbalances will combine with the natural fluctuations in hormones that take place during menopause. The result will be the symptoms that we recognize as hot flashes, loss of memory, emotional imbalance, weight gain, urinary infections, vaginal dryness, loss of sexual desire, and sleep problems.

What's the best way to prepare for menopause and prevent these imbalances from happening? The most important thing is to prevent Pitta and Vata imbalances from developing and to keep the body free of ama before menopause begins. Not all women will experience the same symptoms. Some will have more hot flashes, some more mood swings, others memory problems, and yet others a loss of libido. Very few will have all the symptoms. And some women will have no symptoms at all.

In her book *The Ageless Woman: Natural Health and Beauty After Forty with Maharishi Ayurveda,* noted women's health expert Nancy Lonsdorf, M.D., summarizes three basic types of menopausal imbalances relating to each of the three doshas. These are:

- **Vata-type menopausal symptoms:** Prone to nervousness; anxiety, panic, mood swings, vaginal dryness, loss of skin tone, feeling cold, irregular periods, insomnia, mild or variable hot flashes, constipation, palpitations, bloating, and joint aches and pains.

- **Pitta-type menopausal symptoms:** Prone to hot temper; anger, irritability, feeling hot, hot flashes, night sweats, heavy periods, excessive bleeding, urinary tract infections, skin rashes, and acne.

- **Kapha-type menopausal symptoms:** Prone to weight gain; sluggishness, lethargy, weight gain for no reason, fluid retention, yeast infections, lazy, depressed, lacking motivation, and slow digestion.

The reason for the variation in symptoms, even though all women experience the same reduction in estrogen at the time of menopause, is that so many

TABLE 9.6. SPECIFIC RECOMMENDATIONS FOR MENOPAUSE	
Additional Guidelines for a Vata-Pacifying Diet	
Foods	*Follow the Vata-pacifying diet in Table 8.2, page 123, with the following modifications:*
Increase	Increase warm food and drinks.
Decrease	Decrease caffeine and other stimulants, refined sugar, cold drinks, salads.
Other	Eat regular meals.
Herbs and Oils	Take *Maharishi Amrit Kalash.*
Spices	Cook with spices such as fennel and cumin.
Additional Guidelines for a Pitta-Pacifying Diet	
Foods	*Follow the Pitta-pacifying diet in Table 8.3, page 124, with the following modifications:*
Increase	Increase cooling foods, water intake, sweet and juicy fruits (grapes, pears, plums, mangoes, melons, apples), zucchini, yellow squash, cucumber, organic foods.
Decrease	Decrease hot spicy foods, hot drinks, and alcohol.
Spices	Decrease hot spices such as chilis and cayenne.
Additional Guidelines for a Kapha-Pacifying Diet	
Foods	*Follow the Kapha-pacifying diet in Table 8.4, page 125, with the following modifications:*
Increase	Increase fruits, whole grains, legumes, and vegetables.
Decrease	Decrease meat, cheese, sugar, cold foods, and drinks.
Spices	Increase spices such as black pepper, turmeric, and ginger.
Additional Guidelines for All Dosha Imbalances	
Herbs and Oils	Take *Midlife for Women 1* tablets before menopause begins. Take *Midlife for Women 2* tablets once menopause has begun. Use *Golden Transition Therapeutic Aroma Oil.* Take *Herbal Absorb Calcium* tablets. Take *Blissful Joy* tablets and use *Blissful Joy Therapeutic Aroma Oil Blend.* Take *Maharishi Amrit Kalash.*

other factors are at play. If someone is of Pitta constitution, or if they are eating foods that cause a Pitta imbalance or living a lifestyle that creates those imbalances, they experience more Pitta-related symptoms such as hot flashes and mood swings. On the other hand, if a person has a Vata imbalance due to having more Vata in their constitution or eating more Vata foods and living a Vata aggravating lifestyle, then they will experience more Vata-related symptoms, such as memory loss and vaginal dryness. The same is true of Kapha-aggravating factors.

So if you start to have any of the Pitta-, Vata-, or Kapha-based problems of menopause, be sure to follow the corresponding dosha-pacifying program. In addition to balancing the doshas, it's important to keep your digestion strong and free of ama by following the guidelines for your specific type of dosha imbalance and the general guidelines given in Table 9.6.

RECOMMENDATIONS FOR TARGETING DIABETES

The presence of diabetes greatly increases the risk for atherosclerosis and heart disease. For diabetes, the Maharishi Vedic Approach to Health provides dietary and routine recommendations to reduce Kapha, which is considered the primary dosha imbalance leading to excessively high blood sugar, and to enhance the production of ojas. With increased ojas comes an increase in the body's intelligence in proper metabolism and organ functioning such as the pancreas and the liver, two important organs involved in proper regulation of blood

TABLE 9.7. SPECIFIC RECOMMENDATIONS FOR DIABETES	
Foods	*Follow guidelines for a Kapha-pacifying diet (see Table 8.4, page 125) with the following modifications:*
Increase	Eat more light, dry, warm, bitter, pungent, astringent foods, such as bitter gourd, fenugreek leaf, guar, and well-cooked leafy green vegetables. Increase quinoa, amaranth, and barley.
Decrease	Reduce sweet, sour, salty tastes. Avoid fatty foods. Do not overeat. Avoid heavy foods such as meats, cheeses, and other hard-to-digest dairy products. Avoid ice-cold drinks and foods.
Other	Drink lots of warm water throughout the day to help flush toxins that can inhibit the function of the liver and pancreas. Avoid fasting or skipping meals.
Herbs, Oils, Spices, and Teas	Take *Glucostat* herbal formula to help normalize sugar metabolism. Cook with *Kapha Churna* or sprinkle it on foods. Include the herbs turmeric, cumin, coriander, and fenugreek. Drink *Be Trim Tea* and/or *Kapha Tea*. May use the sugar-free formulation of *Maharishi Amrit Kalash*.

sugar and insulin. Be sure to consult with your physician regarding integrating these suggestions with your conventional treatment plan.

ADJUNCTS TO THE DIET

In the preceding tables, specific herbal mixtures are recommended for specific dosha imbalances and conditions. However, there is one herbal formulation that is highly recommended for everyone: Maharishi Amrit Kalash (MAK).

Maharishi Amrit Kalash: The Most Powerful Herbal Antioxidant

Amrit Kalash means "nectar of immortality." For thousands of years, the formulation has been recommended for its overall disease-preventing and health-promoting qualities. Amrit includes two formulations: *Ambrosia* (tablets, MAK-4) and *Nectar* (herbal fruit jam, MAK-5). Together they contain twenty-four herbs that are carefully selected and processed so that the mixture is perfectly balanced to support more perfect health.

Inspired by this ancient information, Hari Sharma, M.D., emeritus professor at Ohio State University Medical School, and his colleagues have been conducting extensive laboratory tests on this nutritional supplement for the past ten years. From their studies on cells, animals, and humans, these scientists found Maharishi Amrit Kalash to be remarkably effective in reducing free radicals and oxidants in the body—1,000 times more powerful than vitamin C. As you may recall from Chapter 1, free radicals and oxidants are chemicals that contain oxygen in a highly reactive form. They are so reactive that they can damage fats, carbohydrates, proteins, and even DNA. In doing so, they damage cells, tissues, and organs. Free radicals and related oxidants are thought to be the culprits in most of the chronic diseases associated with aging, including coronary heart disease and hypertension. In fact, the most damaging form of cholesterol is the oxidized form.

The natural antidote to free radicals is antioxidants. Antioxidants neutralize free radicals and represent the first line of the body's defense system against these toxins. Dr. Sharma's studies found that Maharishi Amrit Kalash's antioxidant properties are so powerful that it prevented atherosclerosis and cancer in laboratory animals. Figure 9.1 shows that both formulations Amrit Ambrosia (*Maharishi Amrit Kalash* 4) and Nectar (*Maharishi Amrit Kalash* 5) reduce oxidized cholesterol in the laboratory. Human studies have found improvements in mental and physical functioning that are associated with aging. In a study we published recently in the *American Journal of Cardiology,* a combination of the Transcendental Meditation technique, Maharishi Amrit Kalash, Vedic diet, and Vedic exercise significantly reduced atherosclerosis in older men and women, as measured by ultrasound evaluation of their arteries.

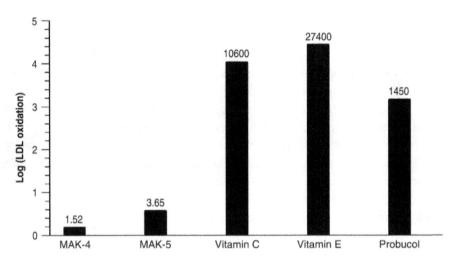

Figure 9.1. Comparison of the Ability of Different Antioxidants to Decrease Oxidation of Human Low-Density Lipoprotein

Source: Data from *Pharmacology Biochemistry and Behavior* 43 (1992): 1175–1182.

How the Herbal Preparations Work

The herbal preparations used in the Total Heart Health program are considered to be concentrated forms of nature's intelligence. Also, like foods, herbs offer nourishment to the cells and tissues and correct imbalances in one's physiology over time, safely, without causing side effects. These herbal formulations are based on the principle that nature's healing wisdom is a precise and sophisticated balance that is preserved in the whole plant, not in an isolated chemical. The sophisticated herbal preparations recommended in the Total Heart Health program have several distinct functions that strengthen the formula. Unlike modern medicine, and even other natural medicine practices, it is rare in the Maharishi Vedic Approach to Health to use even a single herb alone to treat a specific disorder.

According to Maharishi Ayurveda Products International (MAPI):

Primary herbs offer targeted benefits for a specific area of health, such as energy. Supporting herbs reinforce the healing action of the primary herbs. Bioavailability herbs help your body assimilate and use the nutrients. Herbal "co-factors" remove impurities and the toxic byproducts of incomplete digestion from your body. Balancing herbs cancel out any potential discomforts or side effects that can come with the benefits of a particular herb. Together these different types of herbs create a whole that is greater than the sum of its parts.

It is important to use only safe and time-tested herbal supplements. The herbal preparations discussed here have been extensively tested for quality and lack of toxins, such as lead and mercury. The herbal ingredients are employed in their whole component form as foods because it is the wholeness that most effectively restores proper functioning of your body cells, tissues, and organs. This is important because, as we have seen throughout this book, it is the enlivenment of the body's intelligence exemplified in the balancing of the doshas, not the suppression of symptoms that eliminates the basis of disease.

This is not true for many modern medications that all too often cause harmful or even lethal side effects (see Chapter 3). For example, millions of Americans have been using Cox-2 inhibitors (for example, Vioxx, Celebrex, and Bextra) to treat their joint pains associated with arthritis and aging. Recently, however, it has been extensively reported in the medical literature and popular media that these drugs have nasty side effects: they double the risk of heart attacks. Other cardiac problems, such as hypertension-related events, pulmonary edema, and congestive heart failure—related events were also much more prevalent in the drug-treated groups compared with the placebo groups in scientific studies of these modern drugs.

In the Total Heart Health program, herbs and herbal supplements are used in relatively small quantities as adjuncts to the diet. This has proven to be the safest and most natural method of supplement use. The Total Heart Health program utilizes the ancient understanding of how to use herbal formulas for holistic balancing effects for a patient. We recommend that you use products from MAPI because they are based on this comprehensive understanding and are therefore safe and effective. For more advanced herbal supplement recommendations, please consult a Maharishi Vedic physician or healthcare professional. See the Resources section for more information on the availability of consultations and the herbal supplements.

Excited by earlier research findings showing the ability of Maharishi Amrit Kalash to prevent the oxidation of cholesterol and reverse atherosclerosis in the laboratory, scientists at the Institute for Natural Medicine and Prevention at Maharishi University of Management and collaborators are conducting a randomized-controlled study of Maharishi Amrit Kalash, sponsored by the National Institutes of Health, to evaluate effects of the antioxidant on atherosclerosis and risk factor levels in men and women at high risk for heart disease. While this study is not yet complete, the available scientific evidence combined with time-tested clinical experience suggests that taking Maharishi Amrit Kalash on a daily basis may help prevent the buildup of plaque that clogs the arteries and that is associated with atherosclerosis and heart disease. Furthermore, it may help you to live longer with better overall mind and body health.

CHAPTER 10

Heart-Healthy Meals and Snacks

AS YOU NOW KNOW, DIET PLAYS A MAJOR ROLE in the prevention and treatment of heart disease and its risk factors. This is because the purpose of diet is not just to provide fuel, mortar, and bricks for the body. It is to put the mind and body in balance through aligning your physiology with the unified field and stimulating your system's inner intelligence and self-healing mechanisms. Furthermore, to gain the full benefit of diet for enhancing health, it's not only what you eat, but also when and how you prepare and eat these foods. This chapter presents food preparation. Foods cooked and eaten properly will help balance your doshas, stimulate agni, reduce ama, and enhance ojas.

Such foods as date shakes, sweet lassi, ghee, herbs and seasonings, and stewed apples may be new to you. In this chapter, you will learn how to prepare some of these important foods that are recommended in the Total Heart Health program.

Although cooking with fresh produce and preparing organic, vegetarian meals might take some getting used to, it's not that difficult. It actually takes less time than preparing many meat-based meals, and with some practice, you will be able to prepare delicious, highly satisfying meals in no time at all. An added reward for your efforts is that you will begin to feel and be healthier and happier.

PREPARATION BASICS

A settled, nonchaotic environment is best for cooking meals and dining. A satisfying meal consists of food that is fresh and that has been freshly prepared. It is important to use a wide variety of wholesome foods. Wholesome foods are considered to be primarily fresh organic fruits, vegetables, whole grains, legumes, and dairy. Use sun-ripened, seasonal foods, when possible. Sun-ripened foods have reached ideal maturity for conferring intelligence to the consumer. This is because they have been "cooked" by the sun and are ready for ideal digestion.

Avoid using frozen, processed, and canned foods, which are considered to have lost much of their intelligence and, hence, have lower nutritional value. Also, avoid refrigerated leftovers. They are hard to digest and tend to produce ama, which damages your body's fine machinery.

Essential Ingredients in the Total Heart Health Diet

The following foods are considered essential ingredients in the Total Heart Health diet. We include specific suggestions on how these foods are best prepared. An asterisk (*) following a food indicates that a recipe appears later in the chapter.

- **Grains:** These are a nutritional foundation of the diet. Try a variety of grains for fullest nutrition. Use amaranth, barley, bulgur wheat, couscous, millet, and quinoa in addition to wheat and rice. Brown rice is difficult to digest and should usually be avoided in the diet. Instead, try basmati rice, a whole-grain rice that is naturally a creamy white. Spice mixtures can make grains, especially delicious.

- **Vegetables:** Include plenty of leafy green vegetables in the diet. For satisfying meals, serve a variety of vegetables. They are best served warm and fully cooked; try sautéing, grilling, braising, roasting, or steaming. Spice mixtures also give vegetables satisfying flavor and enhance digestion.

- **Beans and legumes:** These provide the astringent taste and are a good source of protein. Use a variety in the diet to round out your meals. Mung bean dahl* (sometimes spelled *moong bean*) is best for overall balance, regardless of your dosha type. Other legumes according to your dosha type may be prepared similarly.

- **Fruits:** Favor fresh, ripe, juicy fruits in the diet. Apples often need to be cooked. A stewed apple with spices* makes a light breakfast. Dried fruits such as raisins, apricots, figs, and prunes should be soaked before eating. Dates, however, are moist and need no soaking. Spiced, cooked fruit desserts are light and easier to digest than cakes, cookies, and pastries. Melons are best not mixed with other foods; enjoy them on their own.

- **Oils:** Because many pesticides are oil soluble, it is important to use organic oils to minimize your intake of toxins. Cook recommended oils, such as olive oil, slowly on low heat, since high heat changes the chemistry of oil, making it more likely to clog the channels or shrotas. Use oils to sauté spices to increase their potency. Ghee may be safely cooked at higher temperatures than oil.

- **Milk:** This liquid is prized as a highly nutritious, ojas-creating food. However, cold milk is difficult to digest. To overcome the heavy quality of cold milk, boil milk until it foams, and drink when warm. Add any preferred spices such as ginger, turmeric, or cinnamon to milk before boiling to increase digestibility and reduce heaviness. Adding water to the milk (in a 1:1 ratio) and then boiling also aids its digestion. Drink milk alone or along with foods with a predominantly sweet taste.

- **Cheese:** Cheese can be clogging to the channels of the body and difficult to digest, especially at night. It is usually not recommended in purifying diets. However, fresh cheeses, such as panir, ricotta, cottage cheese, and soft cheeses such as mozzarella are easier to digest and assimilate than aged and hard cheeses. Soy cheese may be used as a substitute in moderation.

- **Yogurt:** To enhance digestion, yogurt can be used as a main ingredient in several digestive and sweet drinks. Fresh, homemade yogurt is best for this purpose, since yogurt becomes more acidic and difficult to digest over time.

- **Nuts and seeds:** Almonds, walnuts, and cashews provide additional sources of protein and other nutrients. Before eating, soak them overnight in water to improve their digestibility and to reduce any dosha-aggravating effects. Almonds are best when blanched (skins removed).

Generally recommended seeds include sunflower and sesame seeds. Soak sunflower seeds in water overnight, blot dry then grind them in a food grinder, then sprinkle on top of vegetables or grains for a tasty and healthful protein alternative. Other seeds such as pumpkin or flax may be prepared similarly on a daily basis.

- **Spices:** Spices are keys to good digestion, tissue nourishment, and body cleansing. Proper spicing not only makes food taste good, but it is also necessary for pacifying the doshas and enhancing digestion and metabolism. Maharishi Ayurveda churnas and teas are a convenient way to get a balancing array of spices into the body.

  Sauté spices in oil or ghee to bring out their flavor and to enhance their potency. Do not overheat or burn the oil while sautéing. When making churnas or using a spice in its powdered or ground form, it is best to begin with the whole spice, such as fresh ginger, or whole black pepper, cumin seeds, and mustard seeds, and to grind them yourself. When using both whole spices and powdered spices in a recipe, sauté the whole spices first until they turn light brown or, in the case of mustard seeds, until they pop. Then, add the powdered spices, such as ginger, cumin, turmeric, cardamom, and pepper. To elicit optimum effects, spices need to be sautéed only for a few seconds or up to a minute.

- **Salt and pepper:** Avoid or reduce the tendency to sprinkle salt on your food at the dinner table. Instead, ancient texts recommend that salt be cooked into food to maximize its balancing effects on physiological functioning. Add salt, preferably rock or sea salt, to the cooking water for soups or dahl, or sprinkle over vegetables while they are cooking. Black pepper is a digestive stimulant that helps the body metabolize impurities. It has heating qualities and should not be used in excess. When sautéed with ghee, black pepper is said to nourish the brain. Avoid the use of powdered black pepper. Instead, freshly grind black pepper for cooking and seasoning at the table.

- **Fresh green herbs:** Since fresh green herbs such as oregano, parsley, rosemary, sage, and thyme are often too heat sensitive for long periods of cooking, add them to vegetables, soups, and main dishes when the dish is almost finished.

The Cook and His or Her Tools

Certain materials used in the production of cookware and eating utensils are safer to use than others; some materials, such as aluminum, may even be toxic. Therefore, we recommend that you select your culinary tools according to the following guidelines. First and foremost, however, keep in mind that the temperament and attitude of the cook is a major factor in the quality of the food. The cook should prepare the food in a happy, settled environment, with good intentions.

- **Use stainless-steel cookware.** Stainless-steel cookware is durable and washable, has good cooking characteristics, and is considered nontoxic. Cooking in a cast-iron skillet is fine on occasion, but avoid all aluminum pans, baking dishes, and utensils. Aluminum toxicity has been implicated in Alzheimer's disease and other disorders, and small amounts of aluminum may be transferred during cooking from the cookware to the food. Also, avoid nonstick cookware, since the chemicals in the nonstick coating may also be transferred to the food during cooking. Ceramic and glass cookware may also be used.

- **Serve food on china or stainless-steel dishes.** China, either porcelain or earthenware, and stainless steel are considered the purest common materials for tableware. Avoid plastic dishes and utensils. Toxic chemicals in plastics can leach out of plastic ware and into the food. Paper plates and cups are fine for picnics and parties.

- **Use flame heat to cook food whenever possible.** Flame heat, generated by burning gas, wood, or other naturally combustible substances, is considered the most natural and safest form of heat. Cooking using electric stovetops or electric ovens is not as highly recommended. Microwave cooking should be avoided. Traditional experts in Vedic health care consider that the microwave disruption of the food molecules reduces the nutritional value of the food. Cook foods more slowly over lower heat to maintain the food's intelligence and its nutritional properties. High heat can transform chemicals in food into toxic byproducts. Avoid using microwave ovens.

TOTAL HEART HEALTH RECIPES

In this section, you'll find a few recipes for heart-healthy dishes. All of these foods are staples in the Total Heart Health diet and should be consumed often or as recommended in the tables in Chapter 9.

HEART-HEALTHY SPICE MIXTURE

Spice mixtures are often used for stimulating digestion and pacifying the doshas. The following blend of spices can be mixed into cooked vegetables, soups, or grains.

1 part ground turmeric	3 parts ground coriander
2 parts ground cumin	4 parts ground fennel

Pour spices into a bowl and blend well with a spoon. Store the spice mixture in an airtight container until ready to use. The spice mixture will stay useable for at least six months.

To flavor vegetables: To flavor vegetables, cook the vegetables as desired. Heat a small amount of ghee or olive oil (1–2 teaspoons) in a saucepan. Add 1 teaspoon of the spice mixture per serving of vegetables. Sauté the spices until the flavor is released (approximately thirty seconds). Mix into the cooked vegetables and serve immediately.

To flavor grains: To flavor grains, prepare grains as desired. Heat a small amount of ghee or olive oil (1–2 teaspoons) in a saucepan. Add 1 teaspoon of the spice mixture per serving of grains. Sauté the spices until the flavor is released (approximately thirty seconds). Mix into the cooked grains and serve immediately.

To flavor soups: Prepare soup according to recipe. Heat a small amount of ghee or olive oil (1–2 teaspoons) in a saucepan. Add 1 teaspoon of the spice mixture per serving of grains. Sauté the spices until the flavor is released (approximately thirty seconds). Mix into the soup just before serving.

VARIATIONS: Instructions above should be used to prepare the following spice mixtures. All spice mixtures may be mixed into cooked vegetables, soups, or grains.

CHOLESTEROL-LOWERING SPICE MIXTURE

1 part dried powdered ginger
1 part ground black pepper
2 parts ground fenugreek

3 parts ground turmeric
6 parts ground cumin
6 parts ground coriander

6 parts ground fennel

VATA-PACIFYING SPICE MIXTURE

1 part turmeric
1 part black pepper
1 part black cumin

2 parts cumin
3 parts coriander
6 parts fennel

PITTA-PACIFYING SPICE MIXTURE

1 part turmeric
1 part black pepper
1 part black cumin

2 parts cumin
3 parts coriander
6 parts fennel

KAPHA-PACIFYING SPICE MIXTURE

1 part turmeric
1 part black pepper
1 part cumin

1 part coriander
6 parts fennel
1 part black cumin

MENTAL STRESS-RELIEF SPICE MIXTURE

1 part turmeric	1 part coriander
1 part fenugreek	1 part black pepper
1 part cumin	10 parts fennel

EMOTIONAL STRESS-RELIEF SPICE MIXTURE

1 part ground black pepper	2 parts ground cumin
1 part ground dried ginger	2 parts ground turmeric
2 parts ground coriander	1 part crushed black cumin (the cumin is for women only)

STEWED APPLE

Stewed apple makes a heart-healthy breakfast. The addition of prunes, figs, dates, and raisins is a tasty way to start the day and enhance elimination.

YIELD: 1–2 SERVINGS

1 organic fresh, sweet, ripe apple,
peeled and chopped

$1/3$ cup spring or purified water

1 date, chopped

2–4 prunes, chopped

2 tablespoons raisins

1 fig, chopped

$1/4$ teaspoon of ground cinnamon, coriander, cloves,
or cardamom, or a combination of these spices

Place chopped apple in a small saucepan and add water to cover. Cook over low heat until fruit is tender (about five minutes). Add preferred spice. Serve warm.

VARIATION: In place of the apple, use an organic fresh, sweet, ripe pear or a combination of apple and pear.

DIGESTIVE LASSI

Digestive lassi taken with or before meal eases digestion.
Prepared this way, yogurt is easily digested and assimilated.
It's best to use fresh yogurt whenever possible.

YIELD: 4 CUPS

1 cup fresh yogurt

3 cups spring or purified water

Pinch each of ground ginger, ground cumin,
sea salt, and ground black pepper

Combine all ingredients in a blender, and blend on high speed
for two minutes. Serve at room temperature with or before lunch.

HOMEMADE BUTTERMILK

This yogurt drink is recommended in some dosha-pacifying diets
to aid food assimilation and smooth digestion. It's best to
use fresh yogurt whenever possible. For this recipe, it
is important for the yogurt and water to be cold.

YIELD: 1 SERVING

$^3/_4$ cup cold spring or purified water

$^1/_4$ cup cold fresh yogurt

$^1/_4$ teaspoon ground cumin

$^1/_4$ teaspoon cilantro leaf, chopped

1 pinch rock salt or sea salt

Pour yogurt into the blender, and blend on low speed for three to
five minutes. Add water and blend on low speed for an additional
three to five minutes. Skim off fatty foam that rises to the top of the
mixture and discard. Continue to blend, stopping to skim off any
additional fatty foam that develops, until the mixture is watery
but cloudy. Pour into a serving glass. Add spices, and stir briefly
with a spoon. Serve at room temperature.

SWEET LASSI

Sweet lassi is a refreshing yogurt drink that can be served at lunchtime or for a midday snack. It's best to use fresh yogurt whenever possible.

YIELD: 4 CUPS

1 cup fresh yogurt

3 cups spring or purified water

Cane sugar, honey, or date sugar to taste

1–2 drops rose water

Spice to taste (ground cardamom, cinnamon, coriander, or cloves, or a combination of these spices)

Combine all ingredients in a blender, and blend on high speed for two minutes. Serve at room temperature with lunch or for a sweet snack in the afternoon.

DATE MILK SHAKE

This delicious snack satisfies sugar cravings.

YIELD: 1 SERVING

1 cup whole organic milk

4–5 whole pitted dates*

2 pinches powdered cardamom or cinnamon

* Medjool dates make the best shakes.

Boil milk until it foams, but do not let it scorch. Turn off heat, and allow milk to cool slightly. Pour warm milk, dates, and spices in blender. Blend at high speed until dates are finely ground. Pour into a serving glass and drink while warm.

VARIATION: For a cooling, soothing, and nourishing drink, try a mango milk shake. Peel one-half ripened mango and cut the flesh into a blender. Add enough milk to cover the mango and puree until smooth. Add the remaining milk and blend for 15 seconds. Serves two.

NUTRITIOUS RICE

*Grains are recommended in almost all dosha-pacifying diets.
Rice is a sweet-tasting grain that makes a nutty-flavored
side dish for vegetables and soups. Basmati rice is a
flavorful variety of naturally white whole-grain rice.*

YIELD: 2–3 SERVINGS

1 cup spring or purified water
$\frac{1}{2}$ cup organic white rice, rinsed
$\frac{1}{2}$ teaspoon ghee

Bring water to boil over medium heat in a medium-sized saucepan.
Add rice and ghee; stir. Turn heat to low and cover. Simmer for fifteen
to twenty minutes (cooking times may vary; check directions on
package). Remove from heat when rice is tender and the water is
absorbed. Allow to sit covered for five minutes.

To flavor the rice: Heat 1–2 teaspoons of ghee in a saucepan. Add
1 teaspoon of the recommended spice mixture per serving of rice.
Sauté the spices until the flavor is released (approximately thirty
seconds). Pour spice mixture over rice and gently stir.

BASIC MUNG DAHL DISH

*Split mung dahl—which is available at most natural-food and health-food
stores—makes for a healthy, highly digestible, and savory side dish.
Easy to prepare, it can be served alongside grains and vegetables,
or accompanied by chapatis (see recipe, page 160).*

YIELD: 2–3 SERVINGS

3 cups spring or purified water
$\frac{1}{2}$ cup organic split mung dahl,
rinsed and sorted

1 teaspoon ghee

1 teaspoon churna* or dosha-pacifying spice mixture*

*The churna or spice mixture you use for this recipe depends on which
dosha-pacifying diet you are following. In place of the churna, you can
use a prescribed spice mixture, if desired.

In a medium-sized saucepan, bring water to a boil. Add dahl to boiling water, and stir. Boil for twenty to thirty minutes until dahl is soft and tender. Meanwhile, heat ghee in a skillet, add churna, and sauté for thirty seconds until churna gives off a flavorful aroma. (Do not scorch or overcook churna.) Pour sautéed churna over dahl. Stir and cover the dahl. Remove from heat, and allow to stand for five minutes before serving.

SPICY DAHL SOUP

Split mung dahl also makes for a hearty, savory soup.

YIELD: 4–6 SERVINGS

1 cup organic split mung dahl, rinsed and sorted

6 cups spring or purified water

2 teaspoons ground coriander

2 teaspoons peeled and minced fresh ginger root

1 teaspoon salt

2 tablespoons ghee or olive oil

1 teaspoon cumin seeds

1 teaspoon black mustard seeds

1 teaspoon ground turmeric

4 tablespoons coarsely chopped fresh cilantro, as garnish

Combine beans, water, coriander, ginger, and salt in a large pot. (Set aside the cumin seeds, mustard seeds, and turmeric.) Bring to a boil over high heat, stirring occasionally. Reduce heat to medium, and cook for thirty minutes, or until the dahl is soft and tender. Stir occasionally to prevent sticking, and add water as needed to maintain soupy consistency. Remove from heat and allow to cool slightly. Whip mixture with a wire whisk until the soup is creamy smooth. Meanwhile, heat ghee in a small saucepan. Add the cumin and mustard seeds. (Seeds pop when cooked so keep the pan covered.) Sauté until the seeds turn brown.

Pour seeds into the soup. Stir in the turmeric, and garnish with cilantro. Serve warm.

VARIATION: Vary the spices used and/or add your favorite cooked vegetables to the soup.

CHAPATIS (PAN BREAD)

Satisfying and nutritious, chapatis are a great complement to any meal.
Chapati flour is available at natural foods or specialty stores.

YIELD: 4 PIECES OF FLAT BREAD

1 cup chapatti flour

2 teaspoons ghee

$1/4$ teaspoon salt

$1/4$ cup whole cumin seeds (optional)

$1/4$ teaspoon organic baking powder

$1/3$ cup plus 2 teaspoons warm spring
or purified water (not distilled)

4 teaspoons ghee (for frying)

In a mixing bowl, combine flour and 2 teaspoons of ghee; mix with fingers. Add salt, cumin seeds (if desired), and baking powder. Knead mixture until dough is smooth and even. Cover with clean cloth, and let sit for about ten minutes. Divide dough into four balls. On a floured surface, flatten each ball into a flat circle (about 5 inches in diameter). Heat frying pan over medium heat. Add 1 teaspoon of ghee, and fry both sides of the bread over low heat until light brown. While frying, press bread with spatula to make it puffy. Repeat with remaining dough. Serve bread warm alongside the main course.

RICE & BEAN BOTTLED LUNCH

The Rice & Bean Bottled Lunch is for those people whose schedules
don't always allow enough time for well-cooked, balanced meals.
This portable lunch takes minimal preparation time at home,
and the rest of the cooking happens inside the thermos.
For best results, use a well-sealed, stainless-steel
thermos with one-quart capacity.

YIELD: 1 SERVING

$1/4$ cup organic split mung beans, rinsed

$1/4$ cup organic rice, rinsed (white basmati rice recommended)

1–1 ½ cups fresh, organic vegetables,
cut into bite-sized pieces

1 tablespoon ghee

2 cups spring or purified water

1 teaspoon churna* or dosha-pacifying spice mixture*

* The churna or dosha-pacifying spice mixture you use for this recipe depends on which dosha-pacifying diet you are following. You can also use a combination of whole or ground spices to taste.

Heat ghee in a saucepan, and quickly sauté the spices. Add the beans, rice, and chopped vegetables. Cover with water, and simmer for at least five minutes (certain vegetables may need to cook for up to ten minutes). While still boiling, carefully and quickly pour the mixture into a one-quart thermos using a stainless-steel ladle. Do not allow the mixture to cool. Quickly screw the cap on the thermos, and do not open for at least four hours; the beans, rice, and vegetables need this time to finish cooking. For example, if you fill the thermos at 8 A.M., the Rice & Bean Bottled Lunch will be ready to eat by noon.

KANJI WATER

A warm, nutritious drink, Kanji water is especially useful if you are ill, such as with a cold or flu or have little or no appetite. It is an excellent source of instant nutrition when your body is depleted for any reason. Kanji water can be used as a meal replacement if you are trying to lose weight or as a satisfying snack during the day. Kanji water is classically said to balance all three doshas.

YIELD: 1 SERVING

3 ½ cups spring or purified water

¼ cup organic basmati rice, rinsed

1 pinch each of ginger, ground cumin, and salt

Combine water and rice in a pot and bring to a boil. Boil in a covered pot over low heat for one hour or until the rice swells and breaks. Stir well. Remove from heat, and strain out large pieces of rice. Add ginger, cumin, and salt. Pour into a thermos, and drink throughout the day.

HERBAL SPICE WATERS

*Water is essential for your body's structures and functions yet,
when properly prepared and absorbed by the body, it has several
healing qualities. Water helps to remove fatigue, enhances skin glow,
prevents constipation, increases stamina, enhances satisfaction
and contentment, helps digestion, and is cooling. Below are
recipes for herbal waters to balance each of the three doshas.*

VATA-BALANCING WATER

YIELD: 1 SERVING

2 quarts spring or purified water
3 leaves fresh mint
$\frac{1}{2}$ teaspoon fennel seeds
$\frac{1}{4}$ teaspoon marshmallow root

Boil water for five minutes. Take it off the heat and add mint leaves,
fennel seeds, and marshmallow root. Place the water in a thermos.
Sip it throughout the day at a warm but not hot temperature.

PITTA-BALANCING WATER

YIELD: 1 SERVING

2 quarts spring or purified water
2 rose buds
1 clove bud
$\frac{1}{4}$ teaspoon fennel seeds

Boil water for two minutes. Take it off the heat and add fennel seeds,
rose buds, and clove. Store it hot inside a thermos, but before drinking
pour it into a cup and let it cool to room temperature in summer. In
winter, it can be slightly warmer. Sip throughout the day.

KAPHA-BALANCING WATER

YIELD: 1 SERVING

2 quarts spring or purified water
3 holy basil leaves
2 thin slices fresh ginger
$\frac{1}{2}$ teaspoon fennel
$\frac{1}{4}$ teaspoon cumin

Boil water for five minutes. Take it off the heat and add holy basil leaves, slices of fresh ginger, cumin, and fennel. Place the water and spices in a thermos, and sip the water at a hot or warm temperature throughout the day.

HERBAL BRAIN WATER

YIELD: 1 SERVING

2 quarts spring or purified water
1 *Worry-Free* tea bag
1 teaspoon fennel seeds
2 peppermint leaves

Boil water and add tea bag, peppermint leaves, and fennel seeds. Steep five to ten minutes. Sip throughout the day.

HERBAL WATER FOR WEIGHT REDUCTION

This recipe helps to balance digestion, assimilation and fat metabolism for normalization of weight.

YIELD: 1 SERVING

1 quart spring or purified water
1 part fennel
1 part coriander
2 parts licorice
2 parts fenugreek

Boil water, pour in thermos, and add herbs. Drink throughout the day.

HOMEMADE YOGURT

Freshly prepared yogurt that is consumed within a day or two is considered to be quite healthy. It is brimming with high levels of beneficial bacteria that help digestion and strengthen the body's immune defenses against harmful viruses and bacteria. Store-bought yogurt is heavy and difficult to digest and contains little beneficial bacteria. Although you can use an electric yogurt maker, yogurt is easy to make at home.

YIELD: 1 QUART OR 4–8 SERVINGS

2 tablespoons of yogurt to use as starter*

1 quart organic whole milk

* Use either store-bought unflavored yogurt or yogurt saved from a previous homemade batch.

Allow yogurt starter to reach room temperature. Boil milk until it foams. Remove from heat, and allow to cool to about 100°F/40°C). Pour milk into a thoroughly cleaned glass jar or ceramic bowl. Mix in the yogurt starter. Cover the jar or bowl, and set aside in a warm place (for example, on the stovetop or in the oven heated only by the oven light). This gentle heat will activate the yogurt-making process. Let sit overnight at room temperature. In the morning, you'll have delicious, sweet-tasting, fresh yogurt. Consume every day.

POPPY SEED CHUTNEY

This recipe for poppy seed chutney provides a natural sleep aid that balances both Vata and Pitta in the mind and heart. Eat at night, less than one hour before bed.

YIELD: 1 SERVING

1 teaspoon white poppy seeds

1 teaspoon coconut powder
(fresh grated is best)

Small amount of ghee (clarified butter)

1 part shredded coconut

Pinch of ground cumin and turmeric

salt to taste

Mix white poppy seeds with coconut powder. Add small amounts of water while mixing to form a thick paste. Melt ghee in a frying pan until it becomes clear (cloudiness is gone). Add turmeric and cumin, and mix well. Remove from heat immediately, and simmer off heat until color and aroma change. Add to poppy seed mixture, stir well, let stand five minutes. Add a little salt to taste.

GHEE: THE GOLDEN OIL

Ghee is simply clarified butter—that is, butter with all the milk solids removed. It's a time-honored alternative to hydrogenated oils that clog arteries and promote free-radical damage. While you can make ghee yourself, it can also be purchased ready-made at health-food stores or gourmet markets. See the Resources section for ordering.

YIELD: APPROXIMATELY 1 POUND

1–2 pounds, organic, unsalted butter

Heat butter over low heat in a saucepan. Over the next thirty to forty minutes, the water will boil away and the milk solids will rise to the top, and then sink to the bottom of the pan. When this happens, pour off the ghee—the golden liquid at the top—into a suitable container. Discard the milk solids remaining in the pan. *Caution:* Do not leave butter or ghee unattended while heating. Oils tend to burn and should be monitored while cooking.

ABOUT GHEE

All-natural, salt- and lactose-free, ghee stays fresh for weeks at room temperature. It is not hydrogenated or oxidized, and contains no trans-fatty acids. Ghee is considered an effective "carrier" of the fat-soluble portion of herbs and spices to the various parts of the body. Plus, it's so flavorful and aromatic that you can use half as much as ordinary oils. Spread it on corn-on-the-cob; use it to top a baked potato; sauté spices in it; or pour over hot rice or pasta—its uses are virtually limitless. Because the coagulated lactose (milk sugar) and other milk solids are removed in the process of making ghee, it is suitable for those who are lactose intolerant.

These are just a few recipes for key dishes that will help put your mind and body in balance and restore your heart health. Additional recipes may be found through the Resources section (see MAPI website). And, of course, you can create your own dishes with variations based upon these models and the guidelines recommended in this book.

♥ CHAPTER 11 ♥

Exercise and Daily and Seasonal Routines

BOTH MODERN MEDICINE AND THE MAHARISHI VEDIC Approach to Health agree that exercise is beneficial for strengthening the body and mind, building stamina, and preventing heart disease and its risk factors. However, the Maharishi Vedic Approach to Health promotes exercise in a way that is energizing rather than exhausting, and exhilarating rather than painful as in the popular "no pain, no gain" ethic inherent in many exercise programs. Most important, exercise should, like the other body approaches of the Total Heart Health program, pacify the doshas so that your physiology benefits to the maximum. Along with dosha-pacifying exercise approaches, there are various other activities you can engage in to balance your physiology and promote total heart health. In this chapter, you'll learn about exercise and other daily routines and seasonal activities that are specifically aimed at preventing heart disease. This will provide you with additional valuable tools in your Total Heart Health program.

Engaging regularly in physical exercise can produce an array of health-promoting benefits. For starters, it improves circulation and energy and may help to reduce blood pressure, blood sugar, and lipids. However, if not handled properly, physical activity can also have harmful side effects. For example, every winter, a number of people suffer from heart attacks while shoveling heavy snow. Although you could conceivably choose not to exercise to avoid overexerting yourself, this is not a recommended option. A lack of physical activity or a sedentary lifestyle increases the risk for heart disease by 30 to 50 percent. It is also important for you to adopt an exercise program that is optimal for your mind-body type—that is, your predominant dosha type. Your daily and seasonal routines should be equally suited to your specific needs for total heart health.

THE NATURE OF EXERCISE

According to the Maharishi Vedic Approach to Health, exercise should give more energy than it takes. It should bring lightness, firmness (of muscles), a greater capacity for work, tolerance of difficulties, elimination of impurities, and stimulation of digestion. The ultimate goal is to increase the coordination of mind and body in order to enliven the body's inner intelligence so that you can perform all of life's activities more healthfully and effectively.

The Total Heart Health exercise program differs from conventional exercise programs in several ways. First, based on your predominant dosha, it provides specific guidelines for the type of activity, intensity, and exercise environment that's best for you. Second, the program also makes adjustments for the different seasons for best results. Third, unlike most conventional exercise programs, the Total Heart Health exercise guidelines not only benefit your body, but also your mind. Fourth, and even more deeply, the Maharishi Vedic Approach to Health considers exercise as a means to help balance the body at a quantum mechanical level, that is, to help balance your doshas by waking up your body's innate intelligence. The impact of exercise at this level will result in a series of beneficial effects on your total health beyond the aerobic conditioning and muscular strength effects of conventional exercise programs.

DOSHA-PACIFYING EXERCISES

To determine which type of exercise activities will help to pacify or balance your predominant dosha type, see Table 11.1.

Vata-predominant types are quick-moving people without having much endurance. Often they tend toward fast-paced, vigorous activity, but they cannot handle too much of it without getting exhausted or injured. Therefore, exercise that is less strenuous is best for them. Vata-predominant types may enjoy walking, hiking, dancing, and yoga asanas (postures). Because Vata dosha is cold, this type of person needs to bundle up,

Important

If you already have cardiovascular disease or are over the age of fifty, consult with your doctor before beginning any new exercise program.

stay warm, and avoid exercising in cold and windy weather. Consider indoor exercising at a club during winter. Individuals with a Vata imbalance or prominent Vata by nature need to pay attention to these recommendations to avoid further aggravating Vata dosha.

Pitta-predominant types are by nature fiery in emotional temperament and hot in bodily temperature. Therefore, for them, soothing sports in the fresh air or in the water with moderate levels of exertion are best. Because Pitta types

TABLE 11.1. RECOMMENDED EXERCISES ACCORDING TO DOSHA TYPES

PREDOMINANT DOSHA	ENGAGE IN	MINIMIZE OR AVOID
Vata	Light aerobic exercise and any exercise that brings balance and flexibility, such as walking, dancing, short hikes, light bicycling, and yoga asanas	• Strenuous continuous exercise such as long-distance running or swimming • Exercising in cold and windy weather
Pitta	Brisk walking outside in the fresh air and sunshine, swimming, all water sports, bicycling, tennis, skiing	• Highly competitive sports • Exercising in hot weather
Kapha	Sustained exercise such as running, jogging, aerobics, rowing, team sports	• Exercising in cold and damp weather
For All Dosha Types	Walking, yoga asanas	• Exercising to beyond 50% of your capacity or straining.

may tend toward overcompetitiveness, they need to remember to have fun and enjoy the physical activity for its own sake. Also, they need to avoid overheating (in body and mind) by staying in cool, well-ventilated environments. People with a Pitta predominance need to pay attention to these recommendations to avoid furthering aggravating Pitta dosha.

Kapha-predominant types have strong physical constitutions and are typically slower moving. The image of an overweight sedentary person or large-framed weight lifter comes to mind here. These individuals would do better with exercise that reduces or balances these slower, heavier qualities, such as running, aerobics, and rowing. Since Kapha is already cold and wet, it would be better to avoid exercising in cold, damp environments and to seek out a warmer, drier environment with plenty of sunshine. Kapha types need extra motivation to start exercising to overcome their tendency to lethargy. For total health, Kapha types need regular, vigorous exercise. People with a Kapha predominance need to pay attention to these recommendations to avoid furthering aggravating Kapha dosha.

EXERCISE FOR ALL DOSHA TYPES

The following two exercises are recommended for all dosha types.

Walking

Walking daily for twenty to forty minutes in the fresh air and sunshine is an ideal form of exercise for all types of people, regardless of their mind-body types. The speed, intensity, and time that you walk depends upon your individual capacity and body type. That is, if you are a Vata-predominant type, keep the intensity and duration on the lighter side. Those with a Pitta predominance can strive for moderate exertion, while those with a Kapha predominance may more rapidly increase both the strenuousness and duration of their walking.

For all dosha types, slowly and gradually increase the intensity and time of your walk. If you're not exerting enough, you can exercise for a longer period or with more intensity. Always stop when you note signs of overexertion (described below). If you walk or exercise daily and follow the guidelines above, you will increase your capacity without strain or fatigue.

Yoga Asanas

In addition to walking, gentle stretching exercises called *yoga asanas,* or postures, are excellent for all body types, regardless of age or physical training. Yoga asanas were first prescribed by the ancient Vedic texts thousands of years ago and are said to directly enliven the body's inner intelligence. There has been extensive scientific research on a number of yoga asanas showing improvements in cardiovascular health and other aspects of health and well-being.

Yoga asanas balance all three of the doshas, tone the muscles, and improve flexibility, digestion, and immunity. In fact, yoga asanas not only stretch the muscles and increase flexibility, but they also massage the heart and internal organs. These Vedic exercises are practiced in easy but very specific ways. Therefore, they are best learned from a certified teacher at centers that offer Maharishi Vedic educational programs. There are also traditional breathing exercises or balanced breathing techniques in the Vedic tradition that are often taught along with the postures. These help to restore balance to the mind and body and may be learned from a trained instructor. See the Resources section for more information.

GENERAL GUIDELINES FOR ALL DOSHA TYPES

In addition to paying attention to the primary dosha(s) of your mind-body type, the Maharishi Vedic Approach to Health recommends the following general guidelines for any exercise routine:

- **Quantity:** The ancient Vedic texts recommend exercising to 50 percent of your capacity. This threshold is usually when strain begins (and health-promoting and balancing ends). As you go beyond 50 percent of your capacity, the machinery of your body becomes stressed and the energy of your body will be diverted to repairing the damages caused by straining. Instead, exercise to energize and invigorate rather than to exhaust yourself. Exercising according to your body type for twenty to forty minutes (shorter duration for

Vata, intermediate for Pitta, and longer for Kapha types) most or all days will bring these positive effects.

If you feel strained and exhausted, you're doing too much. So, how do you know what 50 percent of your capacity is? You can continue to exercise until you notice one of the following two signs of overexertion:

1. Difficulty breathing through the nose. If you have to open your mouth to gulp in air, that's a sign that your heart is overexerted, the circulatory system is taxed, and the coordination of heart and lungs is disturbed. Stop immediately and rest awhile.

2. Sweat on forehead or tip of nose. It's fine to sweat elsewhere in the body, but when you notice sweat in these two places, it's a sign that you have overexerted yourself and should stop immediately and rest awhile.

- **Morning is the best time to exercise.** Kapha dominates the morning period (between 6:00 and 10:00 A.M.) when the body is at its peak strength, the weather is fresh and cool, and exercise will be most beneficial. If mornings are not available for exercise, early evening (also a Kapha time, between 6:00 and 8:00 P.M.) is the next best time to exercise. A light walk in the evening is often soothing and may help you fall asleep faster at bedtime. (We'll discuss more about what times of day are best for other activities later in this chapter.)

- **Don't exercise on a full stomach.** Strenuous exercise can interfere with digestion, which in turn can cause ama (impurities and toxins) to accumulate in the body. A leisurely walk after meals is sometimes recommended, but it should not be strenuous or rigorous. Also avoid exercise from 10:00 A.M. to 2:00 P.M., the Pitta time of day, when the digestive fires are burning high and it is time to eat the main meal of the day. Wait about two hours after a full meal. Have a light snack of fruit juice, a cooked apple, or some kind of soupy, warming food before exercising and eat your full meal, breakfast or supper, afterward.

- **Try an *abhyanga*, or special oil massage, before exercise.** An oil massage will tone your muscles, get your blood circulating, and prevent injury or strain. Be careful not to use channel-clogging oils. *Rejuvenation Oil for Men* or *Rejuvenation Oil for Women* is ideal because it contains herbs that penetrate the skin, clear the channels, and rejuvenate the cells. Other massage oils suited for your dosha type may also be used (see MAPI, Resources section). A healthful massage oil enhances circulation and endurance by itself. To learn more about this procedure and where to purchase these products, see "Performing a Self-Oil Massage at Home" on page 185 in Chapter 12.

- **Build up stamina in general.** To increase endurance, try eating more sweet and juicy fruits and proteins such as milk, panir (fresh cheese), soaked almonds, and cashews. If your bowel movements are not regular, add more cooked prunes, raisins, and figs to your diet or use *Herbal Cleanse* tablets. Herbal Cleanse tablets are available in natural food stores or at stores where Maharishi Ayurveda products and supplements are sold (see the Resources section).

Not only exercise, but also the routines for other daily activities should take into account the state of your physiology at different times of the day. Moreover, since your physiology is affected by the season, this should also be taken into account for prevention and health promotion. The next sections deal with these factors.

IDEAL DAILY ROUTINE AND ACTIVITIES

The purpose of the daily and seasonal routines recommended by the Maharishi Vedic Approach to Health is to more closely align yourself with the rhythms and cycles of nature. This will give greater support to your physiological rhythms. It is like swimming with the tide rather than against it. Nature already follows a routine. The sun rises and sets every day as the earth rotates on its axis. The seasons progress as the earth revolves around the sun. The moon also has its set cycles. Each hour, each day, each season unfolds in a rhythmic progression. And each hour, day, and season has its own laws of nature. If you eat, sleep, behave, and, more generally, act and live in a manner that resonates with these subtle laws of nature, your body will feel healthier. After all, the human body is a microcosm of all the forces in nature, so the more you live in a way that attunes your body to those forces of nature, the more healthy and natural you will feel.

The different laws of nature for the different times of day can be described in terms of qualities associated with Vata, Pitta, and Kapha. The early morning from 2:00 A.M. to 6:00 A.M. is Vata time, so that's why it's best to arise sometime before it is over to infuse your mind and body with that light, energetic quality of Vata.

Next comes the more slow and steady Kapha time from 6:00 A.M. to 10:00 A.M. when it's ideal to finish up your Transcendental Meditation practice, exercise, or eat a light breakfast and start work or school.

From 10:00 A.M. to 2:00 P.M., the sun is high and Pitta qualities predominate. It reaches its zenith at noon, and at that time, your digestion can handle a large meal. Then the whole cycle of Vata, Pitta and Kapha repeats itself. The second Vata period is from 2:00 P.M. to 6:00 P.M. when activity of the day is supported. Kapha time in the evening (6:00 P.M. to 10:00 P.M.) is a good time to slow down, rest, and go to bed, because its slow, heavier qualities are conducive to a good night's sleep. By the Pitta time of night (10:00 P.M. to 2:00

A.M.), it's important to be asleep, as this is when your digestive system and other systems need to rest and purify themselves. Figure 11.1 provides a graphic illustration of this concept.

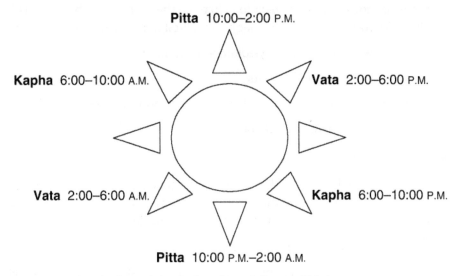

Pitta 10:00–2:00 P.M.

Kapha 6:00–10:00 A.M.

Vata 2:00–6:00 P.M.

Vata 2:00–6:00 A.M.

Kapha 6:00–10:00 P.M.

Pitta 10:00 P.M.–2:00 A.M.

Figure 11.1. The Rhythms of the Doshas through Day and Night

According to the Maharishi Vedic Approach to Health, there are better times during the day for some activities than there are for others. The ideal daily routine recommends activities that will most readily achieve balance of the doshas, and thus restore the connection to your body's intelligence. When you are in this renewed state of balance, you'll find that you are straining less and experiencing more ease and success in your daily activity. Your physiology will be more relaxed, which in turn will help to reduce your risk factors for heart disease.

The Ideal Morning Routine

Rising early and beginning the day with an ideal routine sets you up for a less stress-filled day.

1. Wake up before 6:00 A.M.

2. Empty your bowel and bladder.

3. Wash your face, giving special attention to the eyes.

4. Brush your teeth, scrape your tongue, and rinse your mouth. (Because the toxic substance of ama can collect on the tongue overnight, it's recommended that you scrape your tongue with a metal tongue scraper after brushing your teeth.) This is also a good time to drink a cup of warm water.

5. Perform a self-oil massage, or *abhyanga,* as described in Chapter 12. It's best to wait ten to fifteen minutes for the oil to soak in between your massage and bath.

6. Bathe or shower in warm water to help open the channels of the body. This allows impurities loosened through the self-oil massage to be eliminated.

7. Practice the Transcendental Meditation technique.

8. Exercise or walk for half an hour.

9. Have a light breakfast. (A stewed apple or pear and warm cereal are ideal.)

10. Take prescribed herbal supplements.

The Ideal Midday Routine

The midday routine is structured around work or school activities, and is fueled by the midday meal. Following this recommended midday routine will help you be more effective and energetic in your daytime activities.

1. Midmorning: Perform work or school activities.

2. Noon: Eat your main meal at noon when Pitta dominates and digestion is at its peak. You can take a brief leisurely walk after eating to facilitate digestion.

3. Afternoon: Resume work or school activities.

The Ideal Evening Routine

Early to bed is the key to an ideal evening routine and the basis for the next day's activities. It's especially important for anyone with heart disease or its risk factors to go to bed before 10:00 P.M. during the evening Kapha cycle, when your body is most relaxed and ready for sleep, and before the evening Pitta cycle begins, when your mind and body tend to become more active and when it is more difficult to fall asleep.

1. Early evening: Practice the Transcendental Meditation technique.

2. Eat a light meal before sundown or at least before 8:00 P.M. Sit quietly for a few minutes after eating. Then, take a brief leisurely walk.

3. Enjoy relaxing activities with friends or family.

4. Bedtime before 10:00 P.M.

In addition to these guidelines for daily routine for all mind-body types, there are a few supplemental recommendations to add or emphasize for each of the three predominant dosha types.

Lifestyle Factors to Pacify Vata

- Spend your evenings relaxing with family and friends.
- Be especially vigilant to go to bed before 10:00 P.M.
- Turn off your cell phone when driving, cooking, or eating.
- Focus on one activity at a time.
- Spend time enjoying every day.
- Reduce your mental workload.
- Stop doing work that strains your mind.
- Do mild exercise every day, such as walking or stretching exercises, for twenty to thirty minutes.
- Stay warm and use a humidifier during winter.

Lifestyle Factors to Pacify Pitta

- Avoid emotional confrontations.
- Associate with people who are loving and uncritical.
- Go to bed before 10:00 P.M., after which Pitta increases.
- Plan time to appreciate beauty in your environment.
- Create a home environment that is pleasing and restful to the senses.
- Avoid watching TV at night, especially violent movies or shows.
- Exercise every day to moderate exertion for half an hour or so, but avoid exerting in the noonday sun.
- Choose cooling sports such as swimming.
- Keep your living environment cool, especially at night.
- Drink plenty of pure water throughout the day.

Lifestyle Factors to Pacify Kapha

- Wake up early, well before 6:00 A.M.
- Avoid daytime napping.
- Exercise vigorously for half an hour or more daily.
- Try new activities in your free time.
- Stay warm and dry during the rainy and cool seasons.

BALANCING ACTIVITY WITH REST

Proper sleep and rest are fundamental to good health. Like modern medicine, the Maharishi Vedic Approach to Health recognizes the importance of sleep as a means for refreshing the mind and body and preventing illness. Loss of sleep, inadequate sleep, or poor-quality sleep can lead to reduced energy and productivity, reduced mental capacity, lack of focus, impaired digestion, and dulled emotions. The long-term effects caused by a lack of healthy sleep are even more damaging. They can compromise your body's immune function, raising your susceptibility to disease and decreased mental and emotional stability. Scientific studies have linked long-term sleep deprivation to high blood pressure, obesity, diabetes, and depression. Research on longevity indicates that individuals who sleep seven or more hours per night live longer than people who sleep six or fewer hours per night.

Sound sleep is vital for the health of your heart and cardiovascular system, and the quality of your sleep is as important as the length of time you sleep. Insomnia or difficulties sleeping are typically due to a dosha imbalance. The Maharishi Vedic Approach to Health identifies three types of sleep disorders:

- **Vata-type sleep problems:** Difficulty falling asleep may be caused by Vata imbalance or mental stress. People who toss and turn, and are unable to fall asleep because their minds are whirling, have this disorder. It tends to correlate with anxiety, worry, and rushed activity during the day.

- **Pitta-type sleep problems:** Intermittent awakening may be caused by Pitta imbalance or emotional trauma. With this disorder, you fall asleep fine but wake up every ninety minutes with your heart racing, your muscles tense, and emotions of fear, anger, and sadness. Or another pattern is that you wake up between 2:00 and 4:00 A.M., full of energy, and find it impossible to go back to sleep.

- **Kapha-type sleep problems:** Sleeping long hours but waking up unrefreshed may be caused by Kapha imbalance. Sometimes, it's an early-morning awakening, sometimes it's characterized by sleeping in, but in any case, you will feel sluggish, tired, and completely exhausted even though you've had a full night's sleep.

If you are having trouble getting a good night's rest, first try to improve your sleep using the lifestyle recommendations below. If these general suggestions are not enough to improve your sleep, you may need measures that address your specific dosha imbalance, in which case follow the recommendations in Table 11.2.

- Eat three meals a day: a light breakfast, a main meal around noon, and an early, light dinner.

- Practice the Transcendental Meditation technique for twenty minutes twice a day.

- Go to bed before 10:00 P.M. during the drowsy Kapha time of night, so that your mind can settle down more easily. Rise before 6:00 A.M.

- Eliminate or restrict severely your intake of stimulants or other substances such as caffeine or alcohol, especially before bed.

- Wear comfortable clothing to bed. Organic cotton is highly recommended.

- Decrease stimulating activity at night before bed, such as watching TV, office or computer work, or strenuous physical activity.

- Do not bring work-related material into the bedroom. Do not read, eat, or watch TV in bed.

- Before sleep, engage in restful, nourishing activity. An easy walk in the evening is often settling.

- Keep your bedroom dark or dimly lit and not too warm.

- A gentle oil massage of hands, feet, and neck before bed can aid relaxation.

- Use *Slumber Time* aromatherapy or lavender essential oil to allow a relaxing smell to go to the olfactory center of your brain to help induce sleep.

If, after implementing these recommendations, you still fail to get a good night's sleep, try the recommendations provided in Table 11.2 for diet and daily routine to balance the doshas in the three types of insomnia.

IDEAL SEASONAL ROUTINES

Like living in harmony with nature's daily rhythms, the body also has an internal rhythm that responds to seasonal cycles. For total heart health, we need to pay attention to the effects of the seasonal cycles on the mind and body and how they affect the health of the individual. Just as different doshas dominate during different times of day and night, specific doshas also dominate during the different seasons of the year.

Vata dominates when the weather begins to get cold, leading to winter, roughly from mid-October through February.

Kapha takes over in spring through early summer, from approximately March through mid-June.

Pitta rules summer through early fall, from about mid-June through mid-

TABLE 11.2. HEALTHY SLEEP RECOMMENDATIONS BY DOSHA TYPE

DOSHA TYPE	DIET	ROUTINE
Vata (difficulty falling asleep)	• Follow the Vata-pacifying diet in Table 8.2 on page 123. • Include poppy seeds in your diet, either as a chutney* or with an *Almond Energy* drink combined with warm milk. • Drinking a cup of *Slumber Time Tea* before bed can also be soothing. • Take 1–2 *Blissful Sleep* tablets one hour before bed. • May add 1–2 *Worry Free* tablets if experiencing extra mental stress.	• Follow the ideal daily routine. • Avoid rushed and hurried activity during the day. • Apply a little *Rejuvenation Massage Oil* to your hands and feet before getting into bed. • In bed, breathe deeply and easily to help you unwind.
Pitta (waking during the night)	• Follow the Pitta-pacifying diet in Table 8.3 on page 124. • Try a date milk shake at bedtime. • Include poppy seeds in your diet. • Take 1 *Deep Rest* tablet one hour before bed. • Drink 1 cup *Slumber Time Tea* before bed. • If you wake up during the night, have a snack of 1 cup warm whole milk, with a teaspoon of *Rose Petal Preserve;* may also take 1 tablet *Blissful Joy.*	• Follow the ideal daily routine. • Avoid skipping meals. • Make your own massage oil consisting of 1 part *Rejuvenation Massage Oil* to 1 part cooling oil such as coconut or olive, and apply to hands and feet before getting into bed. • Once in bed, relax by breathing deeply and easily.
Kapha (feeling dull or lethargic after waking up from sleep)	• Follow the Kapha-pacifying diet in Table 8.4 on page 125. • Sip warm water throughout the day. • Eat a light, warm dinner (soup is ideal) and season your food with fresh ginger and a small amount of black pepper. • Drink *Kapha Tea* three times a day and *Slumber Time Tea* before bed. • Take 1 *Deep Rest* tablet one hour before bed.	• Follow the ideal daily routine. • Massage hands and feet, especially the nail beds, with *Rejuvenation Massage Oil* before sleep.

*See Chapter 10 for recipe.

October (see Figure 11.2). These dates may vary depending on your geo-graphic location and local climate patterns.

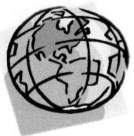

Vata Season
Fall to Winter

Pitta Season
Summer

Kapha Season
Spring

Figure 11.2.
The Doshas and
Their Seasons

Only a little extra attention is needed to maintain the functioning of your body's inner intelligence in accordance with the seasons. The cool, dry weather of late fall to winter increases Vata dosha. If your predominant dosha type is Vata, be sure to be extra careful to pacify Vata dosha with your diet and routine during the cold and dry winter season.

The hot, warm weather of summer increases Pitta in the body. To prevent a further aggravation of Pitta, if that is your predominant dosha type, pay extra attention to your Pitta-pacifying diet and daily routine.

The cold, wet weather of spring increases Kapha dosha. If your predomi-nant dosha type is Kapha, follow your diet and daily routine extra carefully to avoid further imbalances during this season.

BEHAVIORS FOR HEART HEALTH

Lastly, it is important to pay attention to the way in which you conduct your-self as you go through your daily activities and seasonal routines. As you learned in Part One: The Mind Approach, extensive scientific research has demonstrated that your behavior has widespread effects on the health of your heart. In fact, the ancient Vedic texts explicitly describe how negative emotions and behaviors push the doshas out of balance by inhibiting or distorting the free flow of bio-logical intelligence within your body. As an antidote, certain behaviors that en-hance health, happiness, and longevity, traditionally called behavioral *rasayanas,* are recommended. Most or all of these guidelines are found in the traditions of many cultures around the world.

The most important of these behaviors are listed in the following sixteen points. These guidelines are a reminder that you have the ability to choose pos-itive health-supporting actions and to avoid mistakes that may contribute to ill health and unhappiness.

1. Speak truthfully, but kindly and gently.

2. Avoid anger.

3. Be calm and nonviolent.

4. Do not strain in activity.

5. Practice the Transcendental Meditation technique.

6. Be persevering.

7. Practice your religion according to your customs and family traditions.

8. Be clean in dress and grooming.

9. Be devoted to compassion and love and be well behaved with everyone.

10. Be humble.

11. Be respectful of teachers, mentors, and elders.

12. Do not overindulge in alcohol, drugs, or any sensory-stimulating activities.

13. Be positive in all aspects of living.

14. Eat pure foods (such as those recommended in earlier chapters).

15. Keep the company of wise people.

16. Gain spiritual knowledge.

CONCLUSION

The basic yet profound recommendations for exercise and for daily and seasonal routines discussed in this chapter will go a long way to filling out your complete program for total heart health. Remember, all these actions and behaviors share a single underlying effect—they stimulate the flow of your body's inner intelligence. You'll experience the benefits of this effect throughout the day. In the next and final chapter in this part on the Body Approach, we'll explain how you can take advantage of more intensive physiological purification procedures for faster and more potent treatment and prevention of heart disease.

CHAPTER 12

Physiological Purification Procedures

AN INTEGRAL COMPONENT OF THE BODY APPROACH, the Maharishi Rejuvenation Program includes a set of powerful physiological purification procedures used to mobilize and then eliminate toxins and impurities (ama) from your body. These procedures eliminate dosha imbalances and restore the smooth flow of the body's inner intelligence through all the channels of the body, including the cardiovascular system. Physiological purification procedures are recommended seasonally to prevent dosha imbalances from arising and to reverse any imbalance that may have already begun to set in. As part of your Total Heart Health program, Maharishi Rejuvenation is an excellent way to eliminate ama and to strengthen the cardiovascular system, protecting you from heart disease.

At age forty-two, Martin was a busy man. He was running the family's New York restaurant, putting two sons through college, and helping to chair several business, social, and charitable organizations. After a yearly medical checkup, his doctor told him that his blood pressure was dangerously high (170/106) and that he had type 2 diabetes. (Over the past several months, his blood levels of hemoglobin A1c, an indicator of average blood sugar levels, had become high.) Martin started a medication regimen immediately. His blood pressure dropped to normal levels, but he soon found that he became tired and depressed as a side effect of the medication. He tried weaning himself from it, but his blood pressure rose to 160/90 after one week, and he had to resume the medication. His doctor also added medication for depression.

Desperate to resume his normal, full life, Martin checked into a Maharishi Vedic Health Center in his city. There he learned the Transcendental Meditation technique, started an ama-reducing and dosha-pacifying diet, and began a

Maharishi Rejuvenation Program℠, which included specialized oil massages, steam baths, and elimination therapies to remove toxins from the body. Almost immediately, Martin's blood pressure dropped to normal, and he discontinued his medication. His blood sugar tested in the normal range, and he was able to reduce his diabetes medication dosage by half. Thrilled with these results, he voluntarily stopped taking his antidepressant medication.

Completing his in-residence program, Martin continued with regular, twice-daily practice of the Transcendental Meditation technique and learned how to administer at-home versions of the rejuvenation therapies he had been given. After five months, his blood pressure continued to be normal (average 121/79)—without medication—and his blood sugar (hemoglobin A1c levels) remained in the normal range. His depression and anxiety dissipated, and he resumed his busy life.

While the purification treatments Martin received were aimed at treating his hypertension, the Maharishi Vedic Approach to Health emphasizes periodic cleansing of the body at the change of seasons as a way to pacify the doshas and restore balance. Although the body has systems for filtering physical impurities, impurities and toxins (ama) can build up too rapidly for the body to handle, especially at the change of seasons when the dosha influences in the environment change. In addition, after the age of about forty, the body's ability to purify itself by eliminating these residual toxins diminishes.

The method used to detoxify the body is very important. Fasting and harsh eliminative techniques can aggravate the body and cause further dosha imbalances. The procedure for purifying the body and mind should be gentle and balanced. Maharishi Rejuvenation is such a gentle and balanced approach to purifying your physiology.

MAHARISHI REJUVENATION PROCEDURES

The foundation of the Maharishi Rejuvenation Program is called *panchakarma* in Vedic terminology. *Panchakarma* refers to a collection of traditional purification techniques conducted by a specially trained and certified professional Vedic health team. Physiological imbalances may be first identified using pulse diagnosis. Then, an appropriate rejuvenation plan is established.

In this plan, impurities throughout the body are first mobilized by herbalized-oil massages and heat treatments or steam baths. These impurities are then eliminated by gentle heat treatments and mild herbal enemas. This sequence is repeated for several days. It is designed to flush out toxins and nourish and balance the body, leaving you with greater access to your inner intelligence and feeling rejuvenated and refreshed. Implementing these procedures requires the assistance of one or more trained Maharishi Rejuvenation Program technicians.

Other Maharishi Rejuvenation procedures are designed to provide deep relaxation and restore smooth, orderly functioning in the nervous system.

In one such treatment, called *shirodhara,* warm oil is poured slowly back and forth across the forehead in a specific pattern (see Figure 12.1). This is intended to soothe and calm the brain and nervous system. The result produced is one of profound relaxation, mental rest, and brainwave coherence. The latter occurs when the brainwaves in the two hemispheres of your brain are synchronized, a condition that also occurs during the practice of the Transcendental Meditation technique. This experience of deep rest and relaxation balances all doshas, but especially Vata dosha.

Scientific research on the Maharishi Rejuvenation Program was conducted by investigators at the Institute for Natural Medicine and Prevention and reported in the *Journal of Social Behavior and Personality.* In one study, 142 healthy participants received an intervention for seven days consisting of the rejuvenation treatments just described. They were compared with a control group whose intervention was an intellectual description of the therapies without the participants actually experiencing them.

Both groups were tested before and after their intervention. The results of the study are illustrated in Figure 12.2. Those receiving the physiological purification treatment reported significant improvements in general well-being, energy, vitality, stamina, state of mind and emo-

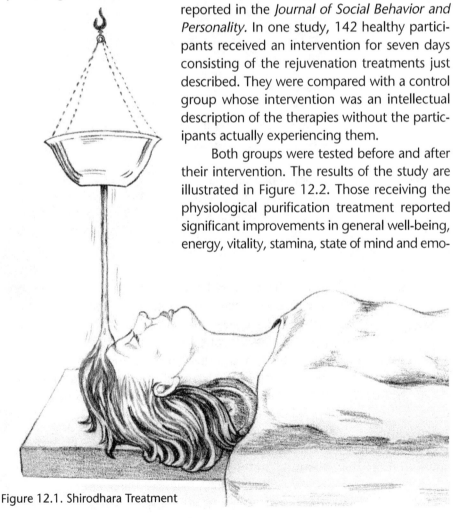

Figure 12.1. Shirodhara Treatment

tions, digestive patterns, and youthfulness. And they reported fewer symptoms from a wide range of previous medical problems. Results of testing using a standardized questionnaire demonstrated reductions in stress factors associated with heart disease, including anxiety, depression, anger, and overall distress. The control group showed no significant improvements.

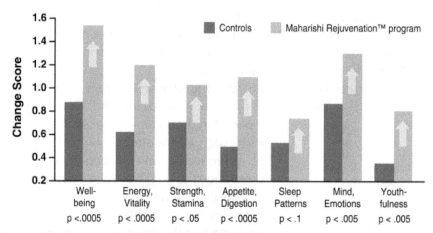

Figure 12.2. Improved Health Symptoms after the Maharishi Rejuvenation Program
Source: Data from *Journal of Social Behavior and Personality* 5 (1999):1–27.

Another study conducted by Hari Sharma, M.D., of Ohio State University, and colleagues at Maharishi University of Management studied fifteen men and sixteen women who participated in the Maharishi Rejuvenation Program for three to five days. The results showed reductions in oxidized lipids, higher HDL ("good") cholesterol, and reduced anxiety three months after completing the purification program.

Another study conducted by scientists, Robert Herron Ph.D., and John Fagan, Ph.D., of the Institute for Science, Technology and Public Policy at Maharishi University of Management evaluated levels of chemical toxins commonly found in the environment (polychlorinated biphenyls [PCBs] and dichlorodiphenyl-dichloroethylene [DDE]) in the blood of individuals before and after undergoing approximately two weeks of the Maharishi Rejuvenation Program. The results showed that there were both long-term reductions of 85 percent and short-term reductions of 45 percent in levels of these harmful chemicals associated with these physiological purification techniques. Taken together, these findings support the conclusion that this traditional, natural purification program promotes detoxification and restoration of the body's normal, healthy functioning in a profound way. The benefits are both immediate and long term. For a powerful boost to your Total Heart Health program, we recommend that you treat yourself to this purification and detoxification program ideally once each season or at least once a year.

Of course, there is at least one simple rejuvenating procedure that you can do yourself every day. That's a self-oil massage, which we describe next.

PERFORMING A SELF-OIL MASSAGE AT HOME

Although physiological purification therapies are usually performed under professional supervision at Maharishi Vedic Health Centers, some gentle procedures can be done at home. One treatment you can do for yourself on a daily basis is an herbalized-oil massage called *abhyanga*. This simple but specific massage is recommended as part of the ideal daily routine to start the day and is very helpful for relaxing and invigorating the body and mind and for keeping the doshas balanced throughout the day. (See Chapter 11 for a description of an ideal daily routine.)

Abhyanga balances all three doshas, especially Vata. The massage typically takes five to ten minutes, and it relieves an array of conditions, including joint pain and stiffness, fatigue, poor muscle tone, poor circulation, poor immunity, sleep disorders, and more.

The best time for an at-home oil massage is in the morning before you bathe or shower. If possible, use organic sesame oil or, better yet, an herbalized massage oil specific for your mind-body type. These oils are available in natural food stores or at stores where Maharishi Ayurveda products and supplements are sold (see the Resources section).

It's easy to set up a simple arrangement in your bathroom that will let you apply the oil to your entire body comfortably. For example, spread a large towel on the floor (or in the tub) to catch any excess oil. Keep the oil in a plastic container and immerse it in warm water just before your massage. You can efficiently heat the oil to a comfortably warm temperature by holding the bottle under running hot water for a few minutes. Alternatively, you can briefly heat the oil in a saucepan on the stove (about one minute), but don't let it become too hot. Warming the oil improves its absorbency.

Sesame oil, which is the most commonly used oil in Maharishi Vedic Centers, has been shown to have antioxidant properties, and is helpful in protecting the skin from free-radical damage. It is also traditionally considered to balance all of the doshas.

To purify or "cure" the sesame oil before using it for the first time, heat it over low heat to 212°F. You'll know the oil has reached this temperature when a drop or two of water placed atop the oil sizzles. Alternatively, use a cooking thermometer. Once this temperature is reached, remove the oil from the heat. Allow it to cool, and store it (in a plastic or glass bottle) for use as needed. Up to one quart of oil can be easily cured at a time using common stainless steel pots. Be sure to observe safety precautions when curing oil. All oils are highly flammable and can cause burns when hot. Do not leave the oil over the heat unattended.

Herbalized massage oils contain a blend of carefully chosen herbs known for their ability to strengthen and balance the body and mind. Specialized herbal oils are available for each mind-body type or for other health concerns such as youthfulness (see the Resources section). So the daily massage with an herbalized massage oil has twice the beneficial power—the benefits from the performance of the actual oil massage and the added healing wisdom of the herbs.

Use the open part of your hand, rather than your fingertips to massage your entire body. Rub the oil in a circular motion over the rounded areas of the face, joints, and stomach. Use straight strokes over the straight areas of the neck, arms, legs, and back. (See Figure 12.3.)

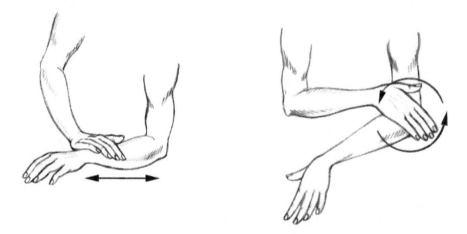

Figure 12.3. Abhyanga Self-Massage

Apply light pressure over the abdomen and heart, and moderate pressure over the other areas of the body. Start with your head and make your way down to your feet in the following sequence:

1. Pour a small amount of warm oil on your hands and vigorously massage it into your scalp. Using the flat part of your hands, make circular strokes to cover your whole head.

2. Move to your face and ears. Massage these areas more gently.

3. Massage the front and back of your neck and the upper part of your spine.

4. Adding more oil as needed, vigorously massage your arms, using a circular motion on your shoulders and elbows and long strokes on your upper arms and forearms.

5. Massage your chest and stomach using a light circular motion over your heart and abdomen.

6. Massage your back and spine as far as you can reach comfortably.

7. Massage your legs more vigorously. Use circular motions over your hips, knees, and ankles. Use long strokes over your thighs and calves.

8. Massage the bottoms of your feet. Use the palm of your hand to vigorously massage the soles and cover every area of the feet. Use a circular motion over your ankles.

9. After the oil has been applied to all parts of the body, if you have the time, let the oil soak in for a few minutes (ten to fifteen minutes ideally). The longer the oil is left on the skin, the deeper it penetrates. During this time, you can shave, trim your nails, rest, or get ready for the day. (You may want to wear sweat socks or other foot coverings if you are going to be walking around your home—both to avoid slipping and tracking oil around the house.)

10. Dab excess oil off with paper towels, if you like.

11. Follow your self-oil massage with a warm bath or shower.

This massage is not only health-promoting but also energizing. It stimulates every organ and revitalizes your skin. It increases your strength and immunity, and detoxifies your body. The massage is a perfect way to start the day and, because it provides daily physiological purification, it is an excellent addition to your Total Heart Health program.

Now that you have become familiar with the Mind and Body Approaches of the Maharishi Vedic Approach to Health, we will move on to the third and final approach of the Total Heart Health program—the Environment Approach. This includes creating a healthy environment and using Vedic sounds and music for a healthy heart.

PART THREE

The Environment Approach

CHAPTER 13

Healing Your Heart Through a Healthy Environment

IN THIS CHAPTER, WE FOCUS ON THREE SIGNIFICANT WAYS in which your environment influences your health and contributes to total heart health. These influences occur primarily through interactions (1) with your immediate surroundings or near environment, especially the homes and buildings you live and work in; (2) with the collective consciousness of the society in which you live; and (3) with the far environment, the sun, moon, stars, and planets. These environments can affect us for better or for worse. In each case, we describe techniques to optimize these influences in ways that maximize your health and allow you to further prevent and treat heart disease. These unified field-based technologies enliven the intelligence of nature in your physiology. This is possible because both the environment and your own physiology emerge from the unified field and are connected to each other by virtue of the field effect described by quantum physics.

In recent years, medical scientists and practitioners have begun to focus attention on the potential impact of the environment on health, including on the health of the heart. Although the medical and scientific communities have yet to fathom this new arena, you can begin to get a sense of the risk factors you face by considering the different types of environmental influences that have recently begun to be associated with heart disease. For our purposes, the following risk factors are categorized according to where they originate in the environment around us:

• **The near environment:** Secondhand cigarette smoke, agricultural and chemical pollutants, and air pollution are examples of external risk factors in this category. In a recent study published in the American Heart Association's journal *Circulation*, scientists describe many of the detailed relationships between air pollution and the development of atherosclerosis. Public health research has also shown that loud noise levels, residential crowding, poor-quality housing, poor-quality work environments, and adverse neighborhood conditions all increase your risk for heart disease.

- **Collective consciousness:** Social isolation, political and economic instability, crime rate, violence, or outbreaks of war in society are examples of this type of risk factor. Studies have shown that during times of social violence, upheaval, or war, rates of heart disease are higher. A greater incidence of serious heart problems has also been correlated with other forms of social distress that occur during times of political and economic instability, such as that found in recent years in the former Soviet Union. Russia is now facing an epidemic of cardiovascular disease.

- **The far environment:** This type of risk factor includes influences related to the sun, moon, stars, and planets. For example, research has been conducted on the influence of circadian rhythms (the twenty-four-hour day/night cycle caused by the earth's rotation) and the seasons (longer-term movement of the earth revolving around the sun) on health. A relationship has been found between daily and seasonal patterns and blood pressure, rates of heart attacks, and strokes.

To achieve total heart health, you need disease-preventing, health-promoting influences from all areas that affect your heart—not only from your mind and body, but also from your environment. In the standard medical textbook *Public Health and Preventive Medicine,* authors Leonard Syme, Ph.D., and Jennifer Balfour, Ph.D., describe environmental influences on health. They state that, "The prevention of disease is a major goal of public health programs. In developing and implementing prevention programs, environmental factors are increasingly recognized as important components." According to the authors, these environmental components include "the air we breathe, the water we drink, and the geographic regions and buildings in which we live. . . ."

Let's take a closer look at some of these environmental influences and the techniques recommended by Vedic health technologies to prevent them from having a negative impact on your health and well-being.

MAHARISHI VEDIC ARCHITECTURE

Public health professionals who study the effects of architecture on health speak of a condition known as the *sick-building syndrome* or *building-related illness.* The phrases are now widely used terms when no infectious agents can be found and some chemical, building material, or design defect in the building is believed to be causing symptoms of illness. This condition is thought to adversely affect tens of thousands of people each year in the United States. Having to work or live in such a building is associated with many symptoms of illness among the building's occupants.

This phenomenon appears to be of recent origin. It was first associated with the energy crisis of the 1970s and is partly due to changes away from open windows and toward energy-efficient living and working environments. Another contributing factor is modern building technology and products, which have led to the construction of homes and offices that contain high amounts of toxic chemicals.

In a recent review article, Carrie Redlich, M.D., M.P.H., and colleagues at Yale University School of Medicine listed numerous negative conditions associated with the architectural environment, including upper respiratory symptoms, headaches, fatigue, skin rashes, lack of concentration, and visual disturbances. According to Redlich, the causes of these building-related illnesses can rarely be attributed to a single agent and often cannot be identified at all, although they are related to some aspect of the building. The Environmental Protection Agency (EPA) projects that millions of Americans will fall sick or are at risk of suffering from diseases due to sick-building syndrome. The EPA has stated that conditions in "sick" buildings "are a significant cause of discomfort and health problems."

Thousands of years before the advent of public health departments and the EPA, ancient Vedic scientists understood the importance of healthy living and working environments. They discovered that in order for an individual to fully experience well-being and total health, it was necessary to live in an environment that was in harmony with natural law. In recent years this knowledge has been revived with its ancient authenticity and is now one of the key components of the Maharishi Vedic Approach to Health.

Maharishi Vedic Architecture[SM], also known in the traditional Vedic language as *Sthapatya Veda,* is a comprehensive, holistic system of architecture and community design. This ancient form of architecture considers the influences of the natural environment, such as the sun, moon, planets, and the cardinal directions on the earth for the best harmony and support in daily living. By living in man-made structures that conform with the natural laws of the near environment, your physiological connection to the ordering and life-supporting influences of the unified field of natural law is enlivened and your health is improved.

Maharishi Vedic Architecture uses age-old Vedic principles of design in a modern setting that integrate the parts and the whole, the individual and the universe, into ideal balance with each other. According to Jonathan Lipman,

A.I.A., former director of the Maharishi Vedic Architecture Consultation Service for North America, "The ancient texts precisely relate specific violations of natural law to specific problems of health. For example, the wrong placement of the kitchen inevitably contributes to weakness and imbalance of the digestive system. The wrong placement of the bedroom contributes to insomnia or chronic fatigue. Therefore, it is advisable to design your home according to the principles of *Sthapatya Veda* design, which always supports and nourishes all aspects of private and professional life for perfect health."

The most important aspects of Vedic architecture that apply to the construction of a home or building include orientation of the building; the placement of the rooms; the proportions and measurements of the building; the building materials; the characteristics of the natural environment surrounding the building, such as slope and shape of land, and degree of exposure to the rising sun; the position of natural elements such as trees and bodies of water in relation to the building; as well as the proximity, angle, and type of man-made structures nearby.

Of these, the factors with the greatest influence include a building's orientation, its structural dimensions, and the placement of its rooms. When these three aspects within a building are in proper balance, the building is said to be in balance with nature and the occupants do not defy or break any laws of nature. Instead of harming you the way a "sick" building does, buildings designed using the following Vedic principles help create health in the people in them.

Building Orientation

The direction a building faces plays a major role in the design of any healthy home or office building. Scientists have long known that animals orient themselves according to various environmental signals such as the sun and the earth's magnetic field. The migration of birds over thousands of miles is one example. Science is now corroborating the importance of orientation in the way humans think, act, and feel. Recent discoveries in neuroscience and physiology show that the brain functions differently according to the direction in which the person is facing.

Deep within your brain is the thalamus. This brain structure acts as a sort of central mediating gateway. It is constantly relaying different information about you and your environment to the rest of the brain where it is integrated into an internal map, so that you can act in a coordinated way in your environment, for example, by not bumping into things. Research now indicates that the thalamus has "head-direction cells" that constantly fire with different rates and patterns according to the direction the head is facing. Figure 13.1 suggests how the direction a person is facing affects the brain.

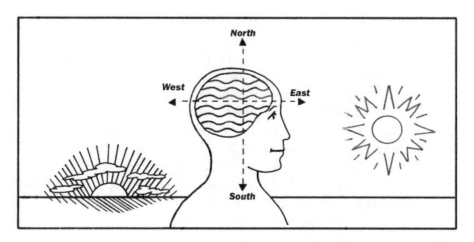

Figure 13.1. Brain Orientation

For the most healthful influence on your brain and nervous system, Maharishi Vedic Architecture advises that a building's entrance face east. This is because the strongest influence on a building is the sun, especially the rising sun. Maharishi Vedic Architecture advocates aligning buildings with the east-west path of the sun to strengthen the connection of the people living and working in the buildings to the larger rhythms and cycles of nature. According to Vedic architecture, the first rising of the sun is the quintessence of all beginnings and its energy is most vital, bringing the greatest benefits to the health of the occupants of the home.

Because of these benefits, Maharishi Vedic Architecture considers the eastern side of your home or business to be the most auspicious place for the entrance. Northern entrances are considered second best. Western entrances are not recommended. Southern entrances are considered particularly inauspicious because they interfere with this natural law and thus can bring negative influences to the building's residents. More detailed recommendations for proper building design may be obtained from an architect or consultant trained in Maharishi Vedic Architecture. (See the Resources section.)

Room Placement

According to the ancient Vedic texts, the placement of rooms within a building also influences health. Each room in a building should be located according to its function so that its residents can take full advantage of the sun's energy throughout the day. As previously mentioned, the traditional knowledge of Vedic architecture relates specific violations of natural law to specific health problems. An out-of-place kitchen, for example, can contribute to digestive problems while wrong placement of the bedroom could contribute to sleep problems, fatigue, or even illness.

Ideally, the kitchen should be placed in the southeast corner of the home. The dining room should also be on the south side next to the kitchen. The study or library placed in the middle of the north side of the house will enhance focus and mental activity. The bedrooms and living room should be located along the west side of the house for more restful sleep and activity when the sun is setting and when the negative influence of the sun has sub-sided. The northeast corner might be used for religious or spiritual focus. Ide-ally, in the center of the building, there is an open area or specially designed atrium that connects all the rooms into an integrated whole. In traditional Vedic language, this central area is called the *brahmastan,* or silent place of wholeness. (See Figure 13.2.)

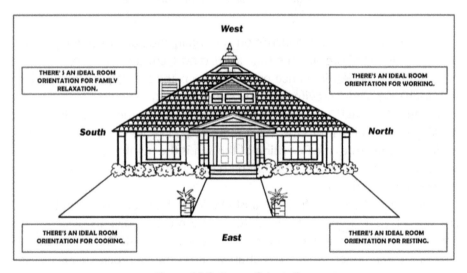

Figure 13.2. Room Orientation

Room Dimensions

Just as every organ and part of the body is properly positioned and precisely proportioned so that it works according to its intended function, so too should rooms in a building have the proper dimensions for their functions to be supported.

According to neuroscientist and Vedic expert Professor Tony Nader, M.D., Ph.D., the patterns of natural law as described in the Vedic literature are repeated at all levels of the universe, from the stars and planets down to the buildings in which you live and work, to the DNA in your cells and the atoms making up your DNA. The same arrangement of planets in the solar system revolving around the sun at the center is repeated in electrons revolving around the nucleus at the center of each atom. The ancient Vedic texts provide for ideal proportions for every room in any given home or office.

Although the scientific basis of Vedic architecture is ancient, modern research methods are currently being used to evaluate the effects of room and building proportions, placement, and orientation on the health, well-being, and success of its occupants. Some of this research is discussed next.

Research on Vedic Architecture

Studies investigating the effects of orientation of buildings on the quality of life of the occupants are supporting the ancient predictions of Vedic architecture. In an analysis of data from 100 people with heart disease, cardiologist John Zamarra, M.D., of Orange County, California, found that a disproportionately high fraction of the patients—50 percent—lived in south-facing homes. If house orientation didn't matter, one would have expected the fraction to be 25 percent for each geographic direction. A more comprehensive follow-up study with 3,000 patients is presently underway.

Professor Hari Sharma, M.D., of Ohio State University College of Medicine describes a pilot study with a small sample of laboratory rats. The animals were placed in cages that controlled the direction in which they slept. In the morning the rats that had slept with their heads toward the north had elevated stress hormones in their bloodstream. The half that had slept with their heads toward the east had reduced amounts of stress-related biochemicals in their blood. This finding is consistent with the ancient Vedic principles of physiology, which maintain that the body is sensitive to compass direction.

A study by Fred Travis, Ph.D., and colleagues at the Center for Brain, Consciousness and Cognition at Maharishi University of Management found that 110 burglary incidents reported in the city of Fairfield, Iowa, occurred in a significantly higher proportion in homes with south entrances compared to those with east entrances. Yet another study, one by Veronica Butler, M.D., showed that mental health levels and financial status among 100 individuals were significantly lower in individuals in houses with a south entrance or who slept with their heads to the north.

When all three main factors of Vedic architecture are present, it is predicted that the effects are greater than with only one or two factors present. To test this theory, researcher Olavur Christian, Ph.D., is studying 100 business establishments in Denmark. Preliminary analysis of thirty companies show that in twenty-seven, the combination of architectural factors described in this chapter correlated with the amount of profit generated per employee of the companies.

Healthy Community Design

Although on a larger scale, the same principles of Vedic architecture used for homes and buildings can also be applied to communities. Ideally, the layout of a community should also have an east orientation. Such communities should also be designed to include adequate fresh air; generous amounts of green space with parks, gardens, and surrounding farms; and nontoxic, energy-efficient homes and buildings. When the basic principles of orientation, placement, and proportion are used to create a town or city, every element of the physical environment supports harmony in individual thinking and action with the laws that govern the universe.

Maharishi Vedic City outside Fairfield, Iowa, is the first large-scale experiment of this sort in modern times. The city was incorporated in July 2001 as a model of ideal city life. It is predicted that residents of such a community will experience greater health, including less heart disease. For more information on how Maharishi Vedic Architecture can be applied to your living or work environment, see the Resources section.

COLLECTIVE CONSCIOUSNESS AND HEALTH

The principles of the Maharishi Vedic Approach to Health are consistent with the principles of modern public health. Both approaches maintain that an individual cannot be completely healthy unless society as a whole is healthy. The ways in which the health of an individual can be affected by the collective consciousness of a society has been the focus of many studies by modern scientists.

One study to produce dramatic results was conducted in 2001 by Ana Diez-Roux, M.D., Ph.D., M.P.H., and colleagues at Columbia University. The findings were subsequently published in the *New England Journal of Medicine* and reported by *USA Today* and the *Associated Press*. The study focused specifically on heart disease rates and the influence the societal environment may have had on these rates. Data for a total of 13,009 individuals were analyzed from four communities in the United States: Forsyth County, North Carolina; Washington County, Maryland; Jackson, Mississippi; and suburbs of Minneapolis, Minnesota. Researchers observed that people living in the most disadvantaged communities, that is, in communities with low incomes and high crime and violence rates, had a 70 percent greater chance of having a heart attack than those who lived in the most advantaged communities. In other words, stressful situations and surroundings in a society can cause heart attacks. Later on, we'll tell you how the Total Heart Health program can reduce this collective stress and thereby cut down on the incidence of heart attacks in individuals.

Correlations have also been observed between increasing rates of heart disease and the effects of violence and war. One study by Dr. S. R. Meisel and colleagues of the Sackler School of Medicine in Tel Aviv, Israel, compared the number of heart attacks that occurred during outbreaks of war in the Middle East to periods of relative peace in the previous year. During the first days of the 1991 Gulf War, the number of heart attacks (acute myocardial infarctions) and deaths increased 58 percent compared with the previous year. Each time there was an outbreak of war, there was an outbreak of heart attacks. This data is shown in Figure 13.3. In the figure, the heavier arrow represents the first day of air strikes and the thinner arrows indicate days on which there were subsequent raids.

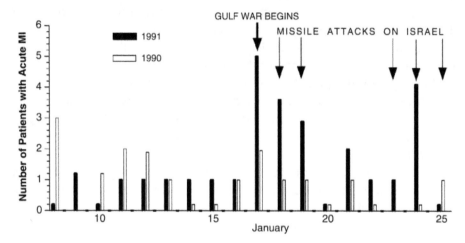

Figure 13.3. Effect of War Stress on Heart Attack Rate
Source: Data from *Lancet* 338 (1991): 660–61.

As a group, the studies show that an increase in social or collective stress experienced during times of violence and war can have a detrimental effect on the health of the people living in these environments. It is telling that heart attacks and cardiovascular deaths in civilians are two common outcomes of a society at war. This finding is consistent with the point expressed in earlier chapters that psychosocial stress is a major contributor to heart disease and at the same time emphasizes the value of a peaceful society for total heart health.

Creating a Healthy Society

Given the dramatic impact that the quality of thinking and behavior of the society in which you live can have on the state of your health, it is important to make your societal environment a positive influence on your health. In other words, by helping to reduce the stress in society as a whole you are helping to reduce your own stress and disease risk. To do so requires the practice of technologies that promote individual health as well as collective health.

According to the Maharishi Vedic Approach to Health, the most effective method for promoting collective health occurs when groups of individuals come together daily to practice the Transcendental Meditation technique and an advanced meditation technique called the TM-Sidhi® program. Remember that practicing the Transcendental Meditation technique opens the mind to the unified field of natural law. This restores the connection of the mind and body to the intelligence of nature. The TM-Sidhi program is an advanced consciousness-based program that has been found to accelerate these benefits. Studies have documented that practice of this advanced meditation program greatly increases brainwave coherence and mind-body coordination, which potentiates other health benefits of the Transcendental Meditation program.

In addition to improving individual mind-body health, scientific studies show that when the Transcendental Meditation and TM-Sidhi program is practiced in a group, the practitioners create field effects; that is, they generate measurable influences on the surrounding larger community. Maharishi Mahesh Yogi, who founded Transcendental Meditation and the TM-Sidhi program, predicted this phenomenon almost fifty years ago. Therefore, it has been called the *Maharishi Effect.*

Even a small group of meditators (equal to approximately the square root of 1 percent of the population) practicing these technologies of consciousness together in one place have been calculated by scientists to generate a powerful and calming influence of coherence in the collective consciousness of an entire population. For the world's population of approximately 6 billion, 1 percent equals 60 million and the square root of 60 million equals 7,746. Thus, approximately 8,000 people practicing the Transcendental Meditation and TM-Sidhi program together in one place would have profound effects on the world. Decreases in crime, sickness, and accident rates, as well as in international conflict and social turbulence have been found to occur as a result of the practice of these programs in groups of several thousand.

Since 1974, more than forty published studies have demonstrated the dramatic effects of the collective practice of the Transcendental Meditation and TM-Sidhi program on the well-being of society. Figure 13.4 shows the results from one of these studies.

Figure 13.4 presents the results of a two-month experiment conducted by Dr. John Hagelin and colleagues on the Maharishi Effect to reduce violent crime in Washington, D.C. Before the study began, it was publicly hypothesized that the level of violent crime in the District of Columbia would drop significantly if a large group of participants in the Transcendental Meditation and TM-Sidhi programs increased coherence and reduced stress in the district by engaging in the collective practice of these programs. This experiment to determine whether more coherent consciousness can influence collective health brought

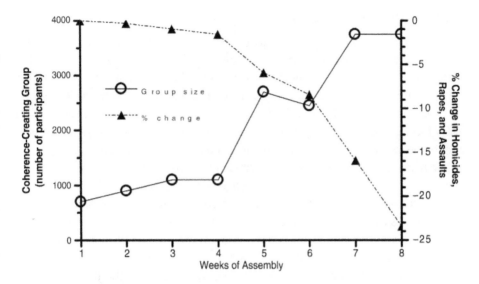

Figure 13.4. Effects of Group Practice of the Transcendental Meditation and TM Sidhi
        Program on Preventing Violent Crime

Source: Data from *Social Indicators Research* 47 (1999): 153–201.

approximately 4,000 participants in the Transcendental Meditation and TM-Sidhi program to the nation's capital for almost six weeks in 1993 from June 7 to July 30. A twenty-seven member, independent project review board consisting of sociologists and criminologists from leading universities, representatives from the police department and government of the District of Columbia, and civic leaders approved the research protocol and monitored its progress.

The key outcome was a reduction in the weekly rate of violent crime, as measured by the Uniform Crime Report program of the Federal Bureau of Investigation. Violent crimes include homicide, rape, aggravated assault, and robbery. This data was obtained from the District of Columbia Metropolitan Police Department for 1993, as well as for the preceding five years (1988 to 1992). Additional data used for control purposes included weather variables such as temperature, precipitation, humidity, daylight hours, changes in police and community anti-crime activities, prior crime trends in the District of Columbia, and concurrent crime trends in neighboring cities.

Analysis of the data revealed that there was a highly significant decrease in violent crimes with increases in the size of the group during the demonstration project. The maximum decrease was 23.3 percent when the size of the group was largest during the final week of the project. The statistical probability that this result could reflect chance variation in crime levels was less than 2 in 1 billion (in scientific notation, $p < 0.000000002$).

An Explanation from Physics

How is it that individuals practicing the Transcendental Meditation and TM-Sidhi program can have such an extraordinary effect on the collective health of a community or a nation? We know from our earlier discussions of the unified field that this unmanifest, nonphysical field connects all phenomena in the universe with the unified field at the basis of the consciousness and physiology of every individual. When an imbalance occurs in an individual's consciousness, it affects the unified field and thereby affects collective consciousness as well. Scientific research has shown that high rates of hypertension and heart disease are all contributed to by stress in the collective consciousness.

The studies presented in this chapter illustrate that when a small percentage of individuals in a society reduce their own stress, they radiate an influence that lowers stress and enhances orderliness and coherence in the society or the collective consciousness around them. In physics, this principle is called a *field effect.* What this means is that an influence in one part of the field can affect the entire field, like a stone thrown into the edge of a pond, creating ripples throughout the entire pond that are felt by all fish and other creatures living in it. When people collectively experience less stressed, more orderly, and harmonious consciousness, the many individual field effects potentiate each other and make the total effect of the group many-fold stronger.

The concept of an invincible barrier protecting society is perhaps best explained by the "Meisner Effect," a phenomenon in physics that displays qualities of coherence and invincibility in quantum mechanical terms. An example of this effect involves super-conductivity in magnetic fields. In an ordinary electrical conductor, incoherent and chaotically moving electrons allow penetration by an external magnetic field. But some metals become superconductors at extremely low temperatures (near absolute zero), where disorder and entropy cease and the molecules become completely coherent (like light waves in a laser beam). Under this condition, an outside influence, such as a magnetic field, cannot penetrate the coherence of the superconductor to disrupt it. A similar situation occurs when a group of individuals practicing the Transcendental Meditation and TM-Sidhi program in a given area exceeds the square root of 1 percent of the population of that area. The participants radiate coherence, which helps to neutralize or repel negative influences in the area.

CYCLES AND RHYTHMS OF NATURE

Medical research has shown that your health is regulated in part by daily, monthly, seasonal, and annual rhythms that are correlated with the cycles of stars and planets in the universe around you. For example, your blood pressure is relatively low at night but rises rapidly in the morning, from 6:00 to 7:00 A.M.

Correlations have been found between this time and spikes in the number of heart attacks in the population. Also, your blood pressure plateaus during the day and then starts to decrease around 7:00 P.M. A corresponding decrease in heart-related deaths has also been found in the population during this time of the day. In addition, there seems to be an influence of the seasons on cardiac deaths. More heart attacks occur in the winter than in the summer.

In medical terminology, these are called *biological rhythms.* Indeed, there is an entire professional society of physicians and scientists called the Society for Research on Biological Rhythms. This society publishes the *Journal of Biological Rhythms,* a publication devoted to understanding these physiological effects on human health. The field of medicine concerned with how to apply the knowledge of biological rhythms for the prevention and treatment of diseases such as heart disease is called *chronomedicine.*

The Body as a Microcosm of the Universe

One recent discovery to result from the cutting-edge research of neuroscientist and physician Professor Tony Nader is that the patterns of natural law described by the Vedic literature show correlations, even down to the level of fine detail, between the structures and functions in the human nervous system and the structures and functions of the planets and stars in the cosmos. These correlations between your inner physiology and the outer environment have important implications for creating total heart health. One pattern shows that the sun, moon, and planets have a one-to-one relationship with specific centers within the brain called the *basal ganglia.* A cross-section of the brain showing the basal ganglia and their correspondence to the planets in our solar system is depicted in Figure 13.5.

As briefly alluded to earlier in the chapter, the thalamus is a collection of nerve cells called *neurons* that occupies a central place in the basal ganglia and in the brain as a whole. It coordinates the sensory and motor inputs that are involved in movement and other vital functions of your body. Structurally, the thalamus is the largest of the nerve centers in the basal ganglia, just as the sun is the largest body in the solar system. Functionally, the thalamus is the central switchboard of the basal ganglia just as all planetary activity centers around the sun. Every one of the other basal ganglia can be similarly correlated with the structure and function of one of the planets in our solar system. Professor Nader's book *Human Physiology—Expression of Veda and the Vedic Literature* goes into this in great detail.

Professor Nader was able to apply this scientific discovery of cosmic counterparts to every level of the human physiology, from the physical form of the body, to its organs, cells, and molecules and DNA within cells. He found that

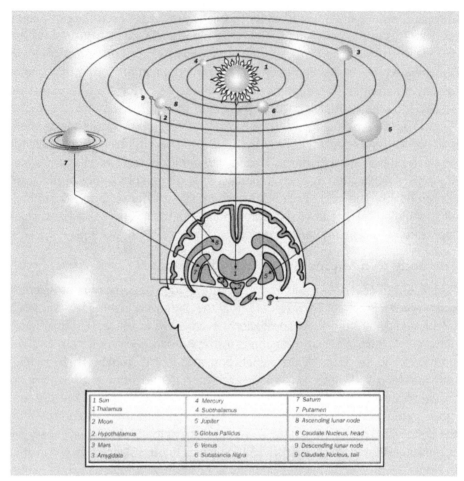

1 Sun	4 Mercury	7 Saturn
1 Thalamus	4 Subthalamus	7 Putamen
2 Moon	5 Jupiter	8 Ascending lunar node
2 Hypothalamus	5 Globus Pallidus	8 Caudate Nucleus, head
3 Mars	6 Venus	9 Descending lunar node
3 Amygdala	6 Substancia Nigra	9 Claudate Nucleus, tail

Figure 13.5. The Cosmic Counterparts of the Brain

the same laws of nature were operating at every level. At the molecular level, for example, Professor Nader observed a correlation between the structures and functions of DNA and that of the planets.

The DNA molecule is wrapped around a central axis in which numerous hydrogen bonds connecting the two strands of DNA are located. These hydrogen bonds correspond to the sun whose composition is 92 percent hydrogen and is the center of the solar system. Similarly, the other components of DNA correspond to the different planets in the solar system. These relationships are illustrated in Figure 13.6. The information in the genetic code of the DNA derives from the combinations and permutations of the biochemicals adenine, thymine, cytosine, and guanine (A, T, C and G).

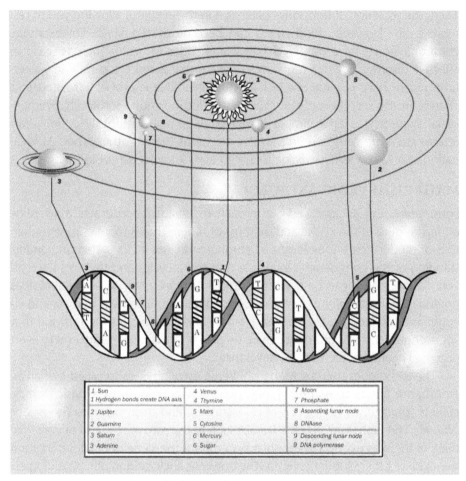

1. Sun	4 Venus	7 Moon
1 Hydrogen bonds create DNA axis	4 Thymine	7 Phosphate
2 Jupiter	5 Mars	8 Ascending lunar node
2 Guanine	5 Cytosine	8 DNAase
3 Saturn	6 Mercury	9 Descending lunar node
3 Adenine	6 Sugar	9 DNA polymerase

Figure 13.6. Cosmic Counterparts of DNA

The fact that the organization of the cosmos is precisely mirrored at all levels of the body from the brain to the DNA suggests that there is a correspondence between the cycles and rhythms in nature as expressed in the microcosm of the human physiology and the macrocosm of the cosmos. This discovery of our cosmic counterparts corresponds to the field of chronomedicine, which studies the cycles and biorhythms of nature and the effects they have on the cycles and biorhythms in the normal human physiology and in disease. The following are examples of how some biorhythms work:

When you wake up in the morning, your blood pressure is typically at its lowest. To get you going for the day, the body secretes more hormones into the bloodstream. By the end of the day, your blood pressure is typically higher.

Then, the secretion of hormones decreases in the evening, allowing you to rest more easily. However, biorhythms can become dysregulated. For example, chronobiologists have observed seasonal changes in health such as seasonal affective disorder (SAD), a form of depression that is more common in wintertime when there is a relative lack of sunshine. SAD is probably related to a change in the secretion of the mood-elevating hormone serotonin. Premenstrual syndrome is an example of dysregulation of a monthly cycle. Heart attacks are more common on Monday mornings than at other times. As fascinating as it is, modern medicine is limited in its knowledge of biorhythms.

MAHARISHI VEDIC ASTROLOGY

Fortunately, the ancient Vedic approach to health incorporates a scientific understanding of the cycles and rhythms of nature that is more complete than that of modern chronobiology and chronomedicine. It is a systematic understanding of the considerable influence that these cycles and rhythms have on your health, and it can be used to predict future events in your life as well as potential health problems. As a science, it contains a systematic body of knowledge; as a technology, it contains clearly defined techniques for applying that knowledge. Most important, it can be used to improve your health and to avert potential health problems from developing.

The techniques used by Maharishi Vedic Astrology℠ (also called Maharishi *Jyotish*) are based on mathematical calculations involving three basic factors: planets (*grahas*), constellations of stars (*rashis*), and their locations (houses or *bhavas*). The grahas are celestial bodies such as the sun, moon, and planets. We think of them as existing in the solar system, but the same principles of natural law exist at other, subtler levels of the universe, including in our physiologies. In the sky, the rashis correspond to the constellations of the zodiac. In the body, the rashis correlate to specific characteristics of individual physiology. The bhavas represent areas of human physiology, health, and activity (for example, education, profession, and family life).

An expert in Maharishi Vedic Astrology calculates trends in the events and circumstances of an individual's life and their timing in terms of planetary cycles. The process involves observing events in the macrocosm (the cosmos) to predict corresponding events in the microcosm (the individual). One can read the story of an individual's past, present, and future from the map of the universe. Maharishi Vedic Astrology can make predictions because the laws of nature that guide the cycles of the stars and planets also guide the unfoldment of your life as illustrated by the discovery of the body's cosmic counterparts. From this perspective, the evolution of an individual life is a localized expression of the sequential evolutionary unfolding of the universe.

The Birth Chart

The basic tool used in Maharishi Vedic Astrology is the birth chart. Your birth chart shows the positions and relationships of the planets and stars at the time of your birth. To create a birth chart, an expert in Maharishi Vedic Astrology uses the time, date, and place of your birth.

The birth chart is like a blueprint of your life. It is analogous to the Human Genome Project, a multi-billion dollar project undertaken by the U.S. Department of Energy, National Institutes of Health scientists, and other researchers to chart the genetic information within the twenty-three pairs of chromosomes called your *genome.* By charting your DNA, you gain access to the blueprint and location of all knowledge of the human physiology. The goal of the genome project was to better understand the role of genes in human health and in the development of common diseases such as heart disease, diabetes, and mental illness, in order to derive new methods for the prevention, early detection, and treatment of disease. However, the genome does not contain sufficient information to predict your behavior whereas Maharishi Vedic Astrology has that potential.

This distinction is very important because, as Walter Willet, M.D., Dr.P.H., of Harvard University has pointed out, conventional genetics predicts 20 percent of heart disease, and lifestyle and behavioral factors account for approximately 80 percent of your risk for heart attack. Maharishi Vedic Astrology provides elaborate and detailed information on health patterns, risk factors, and behavioral tendencies throughout your life—from next month to sixty years from now. This information fills in the missing gaps in modern medical predictive diagnosis.

Based on the configuration of the planets displayed in the birth chart, Maharishi Vedic Astrology experts apply the ancient and time-tested principles from the Vedic tradition and are thus able to predict when and how future health conditions and events will develop in the different areas of your life. With these predictions in hand, you can use the other approaches of the Total Heart Health program to neutralize negative tendencies and prevent ill health, including heart disease.

Our clinical experience has corroborated the ancient Vedic texts in finding that health imbalances that are diagnosed by the Vedic approach correlate with the states of the planets and stars in the birth chart. The movements of the planets and stars have reflected the changing states of balance or imbalance of the three doshas—Vata, Pitta, and Kapha—in the physiology of our patients.

Having this knowledge gives you greater insight into your mind and body so that predispositions toward heart disease and other chronic disorders can be predicted with accuracy. This information can be vastly more accurate and useful than many modern laboratory tests for cardiovascular risk. With this additional knowledge about your health, you can take preventive measures long before symptoms of a heart attack or the risk factors for heart disease occur. Prevention is the best possible medicine for total health. This reflects the old saying "an ounce of prevention is worth a pound of cure."

When performed by a trained expert, Maharishi Vedic Astrology is a powerful method of predicting the health patterns and trends that is not available by reading your daily horoscope in the newspaper or through any other manner of astrology or prediction. It is a mathematically based scientific system that explains how the cycles and rhythms of nature impact the changes and developments in your physiology. This knowledge of the Maharishi Vedic Approach to Health allows you to foresee and avert health problems before they arise.

Maharishi Yagya Program—Vedic Engineering

Another valuable type of preventive measure, one that is unique to Maharishi Vedic Astrology, is a traditional Vedic performance called Maharishi Yagya®. This is a form of Vedic engineering conducted by life-long experts in the Vedic tradition known as *pandits*. In these traditional Vedic procedures, highly trained experts chant different parts of the Vedic literature. As we describe in the next chapter, Vedic sounds used properly can have powerful effects at the level of the unified field to neutralize negative patterns or to augment positive patterns. This is much like destructive or constructive interference of waves described by modern physics. In everyday terms, you can neutralize an oncoming wave pattern using its opposite vibrational values or you can augment a wave pattern by applying the technology at precisely the right frequency and moment to create a matching, supplementary wave.

For example, Mike's yearly Maharishi Vedic Astrology reading had indicated that some chest problems could arise within the year. Mike maintained a balanced routine and was on the look out for any health problems, especially in his chest. When he started having premature ventricular contractions (PVCs), a form of heart disease in which the beating of the ventricle is less coordinated with the beating of the other heart chambers, he saw his doctors immediately. The doctors assured Mike that the condition was annoying but not life threatening. They also told him the only relief they could offer was a beta-blocker that may or may not decrease the intensity of the condition, and there could be side effects from the drug. Mike opted not to take the drug and instead turned to Vedic engineering to help his health situation.

"I had a Maharishi Yagya prescribed to help counteract this problem," says Mike. "The PVCs I was experiencing started to decrease during the yagya performance and two weeks later, they went away completely."

To understand how Maharishi Yagya performances work, think of Newton's Third Law of Motion, the principle of action and reaction, which states that for every action, there is an equal positive or negative reaction. When you throw a stone in a pond, it creates ripples that return back to you standing on shore (see Figure 13.7). You can control the force and height of the ripples with the weight and thrust of the stone. Or when you throw a ball against a wall, it flies back at you. You can divert the ball's path with a racquet or bat to deflect the ball away from you. In the same way, your thoughts and actions create influences that echo throughout the universe. Every one of your thoughts, emotions, words, and actions has an effect—positive or negative—that will return to you in time.

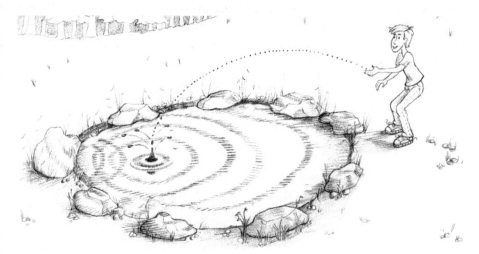

Figure 13.7. Stone Thrown in Pond Illustrating Action and Reaction

Through Maharishi Vedic Astrology, an expert can precisely calculate when such an influence will affect you, and what kind of Maharishi Yagya is needed to avoid future harmful effects. If an influence is negative, and you or someone in your family will face a period of weak health for example, the expert will recommend a yagya performance to dissolve the impact of such an adverse planetary influence. Note that the planetary patterns are just a signpost of the trends in your life. These trends can be changed.

In order for a Maharishi Yagya performance to be effective and successful, it must be conducted correctly. Maharishi Yagya performances are conducted by Maharishi Vedic pandits in India who are experts in Maharishi Yagyas and who have been meticulously trained in yagya performance. There is no real need for the performance to be conducted close by. These experts are deeply rooted in the Vedic tradition and typically come from families where these Vedic traditions have been passed down from generation to generation for countless

years. They perform the Vedic engineering from the deepest level of their awareness, a level at or close to the unified field. Second, Maharishi Vedic Astrology
together with Maharishi Yagyas provides a powerful package of knowledge and
technologies to help avert or minimize illness and disease and enhance good
health.

An expert in Maharishi Vedic Astrology can identify the planetary trends in
your life that indicate the potential for heart disease or its major risk factors. If a
Maharishi Vedic astrology expert predicts illness, you can take steps to avoid it.
If they recommend Vedic engineering, you can have the yagya performed to
neutralize the planetary influences that have lead to illness or may do so in the
future. In addition, you can consult a Maharishi Vedic physician or practitioner
and take steps to dissolve any physiological imbalances that are already there
and that could lead to further illness. To find out more about Maharishi Yagya
programs, see the Resources section.

CHAPTER 14

Vedic Sounds
for a Healthy Heart

SOUNDS ARE COMPOSED OF VIBRATIONS. Sounds are everywhere and they play many roles in our daily lives. They permeate every aspect of the environment, from the rhythm of the beating heart to the trill of a bird, to the radio frequencies present in the outermost cosmos. It's not surprising, then, that sound also can affect your health and well-being. This chapter introduces you to the effects of specific Vedic sounds and how they resonate with fundamental natural laws in your physiology. The Maharishi Vedic Sound technologies described in this chapter use the knowledge of these principles and the specific sounds of the Veda and Vedic literature to transform different aspects of the physiology back to good health. This is a potent new paradigm for creating total heart health from the level of the unified field of natural law.

Research on music has shown that the cardiovascular system and other physiological systems in the body are exquisitely sensitive to different types of sound. Unlikely as that may seem, a number of modern scientific studies evaluating the effects of sound on the heart have found that excessively loud noise, or other discordant sounds in work or living environments contribute to higher rates of hypertension. Research has also shown that certain kinds of music have a calming and soothing effect and can lower blood pressure and stress hormones while soothing the mind.

THE NATURE OF SOUND

It is understood in the Maharishi Vedic Approach to Health, and a verified fact in quantum physics, that as the laws of nature first emerge from the unmanifest unified field, they express themselves in the material world as subtle waves, waves that then go on to create the rest of the material world. From this broad perspective, all matter, including DNA, cells, tissues, organs, and your whole physiology, is derived from the primordial vibrations of natural law emerging from the unified field. (For a graphic depiction of the sequential unfolding of matter, refer back to Figure 4.1 on page 64.) Furthermore, the sound and rhythms of the vibrations at this most subtle level were cognized thousands of years ago by Vedic sages and are available as the sounds of the Veda and Vedic literature. Therefore, the sounds of the Veda are the sounds of intelligence at the basis of physiology and, thus, health.

MAHARISHI VEDIC SOUND THERAPIES

The use of specific sequences of recited or chanted Vedic sounds to directly enliven the body's inner intelligence is considered a powerful approach for achieving heart health. As you may recall, neuroscientist Professor Tony Nader, M.D., Ph.D., discovered direct structural and functional correlations between each aspect of the Veda, or knowledge, found in the ancient Vedic texts and a specific area of the human body. That is, the same impulses of intelligence found in the unified field that give rise to the forty aspects of the Vedic litera-ture also give rise to and are expressed in the human body. Professor Nader's discovery illustrates the connection of the human physiology to the unified field and the Veda, the storehouse for the organizing power of natural law. This means that you have, deep inside you, a blueprint for living perfect health within your body. And you have the basis for a complete healthcare system that affects your mind, body, and environment from the most profound level of life. The health of your body, including your heart, depends on maintaining a lively connection with this underlying blueprint in the unified field.

If this connection gets blocked and the body forgets how to function according to this blueprint, then the wave pattern gets distorted. You lose the connection to the organizing power of nature's intelligence and thereby lose your capacity for healthy functioning. Listening to the sounds of the Veda and Vedic literature can normalize the wave function in specific parts of the body and restore the connection to the blueprint of health within your physiology. The sounds of the Veda contain the patterns that elicit perfect functioning in corresponding areas of the mind and body.

In effect, each part of the body is associated with a particular sound sequence. Any weakness or abnormal activity in your physiology can be cor-rected by experiencing the sounds of the associated aspect of the Vedic litera-ture. For example, if your shoulder is damaged, then you listen to that part of the Vedic literature that corresponds with the shoulder. Or if the knee is injured, then you use that aspect of the Vedic literature associated with the knee. The Vedic sounds help remove physiological obstructions and restore the original, perfect design of the human nervous system. Of course, there are specific types of sounds for the heart and cardiovascular system and for heart disease.

As an example, Hari Sharma, M.D., and his colleagues at Ohio State University studied the effects of Vedic sounds on human cancer cells in vitro. They found that exposure of the cells to certain Vedic sounds reduced the growth of the cancer cells. (The ability to attenuate the unchecked growth of malignant cells is an important goal in cancer treatment.) In contrast, hard-rock music increased cancer cell growth. Dr. Sharma hypothesized that the specific rhythmic, low frequencies of the Vedic sounds may have strengthened the vibrations of normal DNA, while inhibiting the growth of cancer cells. He speculated that hard-rock music characteristically includes numerous high-frequency sounds, which may account for the fact that this kind of music increased the growth of the cancer cells in his study.

Maharishi Gandharva Veda Music

Maharishi Gandharva Veda is the branch of Vedic literature that expresses the integrating and harmonizing qualities of natural law. Its expression in the human physiology is the cycles and rhythms of the body. This includes the heart and the cardiovascular system. Research shows that Maharishi Gandharva Veda[SM] music enhances mental and physical health simply by listening to it for brief periods during the day. It's not unlike enjoying a concert in your living room, but instead of Bach, Beethoven, or relaxation music, you enjoy an ancient symphony consisting of various *ragas,* or melodies, that best correspond to the specific natural laws, that are lively during specific times of the day or night.

In ancient Vedic cultures, where the knowledge of Veda was an integral part of daily life, these melodies were used for specific purposes such as for health or happiness. Each melody expresses the unique impulses or qualities of nature during a specific period of the day or night. The twenty-four-hour day has been divided into eight three-hour periods (for example, 7:00–10:00 A.M.) with appropriate music available for each period. Listening to the ragas brings your surroundings into harmony with these impulses, and helps align your physiology with the impulses of nature. It also helps neutralize environmental stress, and can assist in creating a soothing healthy environment in your home and workplace. All these effects balance the doshas.

In one study, Drs. R. Rasmussen, David Orme-Johnson, and Robert Keith Wallace at Maharishi University of Management evaluated the ability of Gandharva Veda music to promote integrated brain activity of listeners. They analyzed the intensity of various frequencies of brainwaves recorded by EEG. While listening to the Gandharva Veda Music, volunteers exhibited a clear increase in the electrical potentials (signals) within the theta–wave range (frequencies 4–8

Hertz). This type of brainwave pattern is indicative of deep relaxation. A somewhat similar pattern is elicited during the practice of the Transcendental Meditation technique.

There are Gandharva Veda melodies for all twenty-four hours of the day, featuring various instruments such as the flute, sitar (a stringed instrument), and tabla (a type of drum). It is best to listen to the music of Maharishi Gandharva Veda while relaxed and not engaging in other activities such as driving. You can listen as much as you comfortably have time for. The melodies are ideal to help relax in the evening and to help you fall asleep, or if you want to take a break during the day. They are available on audiocassette or compact disk and can be played in the home or office. This music is also often used in clinical settings of Maharishi Vedic Health Centers to help balance the doshas of the guests and to energize their minds and bodies.

For more information on incorporating Maharishi Gandharva Veda music therapy into your Total Heart Health program, see the Resources section.

Maharishi Vedic Vibration Technology

You can listen to Vedic sounds and ragas on an appropriate media such as an audiotape or CD recording. Alternatively, you can utilize another potent form of Vedic sound therapy known as Maharishi Vedic Vibration Technology^{SM}. This therapy uses sounds from the Vedic literature on an even quieter and subtler level.

Maharishi Vedic Vibration Technology works on the level of the unified field that connects you with nature around you. During the treatments, a trained Maharishi Vedic Vibration practitioner, who is knowledgeable in the forty aspects of Vedic knowledge, chooses the Vedic sounds suited to your disorder. The expert whispers within himself or herself specific sounds traditionally used for your particular health concerns and then directs them to the affected part of the body by breath directed to or touching the affected body part. Individuals typically receive approximately three ninety-minute treatments for each disorder. The treatments are gentle, pleasant, and noninvasive. The sounds wake up the inner intelligence in the affected area of the body and help the body to heal quickly. You typically know that it's working effectively because a person often experiences immediate relief from symptoms.

One recipient of Maharishi Vedic Vibration Technology described it as follows: "Heart disease runs in my family. Three of my grandparents died from heart disease and my father, who was put on hypertension medication while in his mid-thirties, had to undergo cardiovascular surgery. I am also susceptible, and if I am not very careful, my blood pressure climbs rapidly. But, by practicing the Transcendental Meditation technique conscientiously, exercising regularly, and following a balanced diet I have been able to stay off of medication so far. Even so, before my Maharishi Vedic Vibration Technology consultation, my blood pressure climbed to a worrisome 150/90 or higher by mid-afternoon. Since my consultation, my blood pressure hasn't exceeded 130/85 and is almost always at 120/80 or better.

"The nicest part, though, is that my experience of life has been lighter and happier since my treatment. The pace of events feels slower and more enjoyable even though my outward circumstances haven't changed."

Two scientific studies on the effects of Maharishi Vedic Vibration Technology and chronic disorders were conducted by teams of researchers at the Maharishi European Research University in Vlodrop, Holland, and the Institute for Natural Medicine and Prevention. Results from the first study reported in the journal *Frontiers of Bioscience* showed reductions in blood pressure and other cardiovascular disorders, anxiety and depression, insomnia, and back and neck pain, among other conditions, with just a few sessions of Maharishi Vedic Vibration Technology. In this study, more than 200 individuals with cardiovascular disease or a range of other chronic disorders received three ninety-minute sessions of Maharishi Vedic Vibration Technology. On average, participants reported 40 percent fewer symptoms, showing that when a specific vibration or sound of the Veda is available to a specific part of the physiology, the underlying intelligence of the body is enlivened.

The second study was designed according to the most rigorous scientific standards. That is, it was a randomized, double-blind, placebo-controlled clinical trial. In this experiment, a single thirty-minute session of Maharishi Vedic Vibration Technology greatly reduced the symptoms of chronic arthritis among sufferers compared with a group that received a placebo. Interestingly, arthritis involves inflammation of the joint tissues, and both modern medicine and the Vedic perspective consider that inflammation also plays a role in atherosclerosis and heart disease. Therefore, the improvements in this inflammatory condition may have relevance for heart disease. This research studied more than 175 participants who had been suffering for years from painful arthritic conditions of the joints or spine. After a single session of Maharishi Vedic Vibration Technology, 40 percent of the participants reported 100 percent relief from pain, even though they had suffered from their disease for an average of ten years. Because there was a control group, the results suggest that the beneficial effects were due to an active intervention and not to a placebo or other spurious effects. Moreover, not only was Maharishi Vedic Vibration Technology immediately effective in relieving a chronic condition, but also there were no side effects.

What in modern science might explain these positive effects of Vedic sounds? In physics, theories of "self-organization" and "chaos" tell us that a stimulus in the environment can transform a disorderly system into an orderly one. These theories show that dynamic mathematical patterns easily shift from chaos to order when controlled mathematical parameters are introduced. Relating this to the body, a study of brainwave patterns showed that a slight stimulus applied to the receptor neurons in the nasal passages induced a major shift in the firing patterns of the brain's neurons. These theories, along with the principles of the Vedic approach, provide an initial explanation of the mechanics by which the Maharishi Vedic Vibration Technology can transform a disorderly condition of bodily functioning such as hypertension or other cardiovascular diseases into a healthier, more orderly one. In other words, a disorderly condition, in this case a less-than-perfect sequence of sounds underlying the physiological imbalance (cardiovascular or otherwise), becomes more orderly with the introduction of the intelligence inherent in the proper sequence of sounds.

For more information about Maharishi Vedic Vibration Technology, see the Resources section.

A NEW PARADIGM FOR HEALTH CARE

The use of Vedic sound technologies for health represents a major advance that, in our opinion, will help shape the future of modern medicine generally and heart disease prevention specifically. This is medicine practiced at a most refined level, at the quantum mechanical level of the unified field. This set of technologies together with the Mind, Body, and Environment Approaches of the Total Heart Health program forms a total package of knowledge and healthcare technologies for the prevention and treatment of heart disease.

🌱 EPILOGUE 🌱

Putting It All Together

Integrating the Mind, Body, and Environment Approaches for Total Heart Health

THIS BOOK HAS PRESENTED THE THREE MAJOR approaches of the Maharishi Vedic Approach to Health for achieving complete heart health, including how they work, what their major benefits are, and how you can get started with each. We discussed the benefits of the Mind Approach and the Transcendental Meditation program for your heart health; the advantages of the Body Approach with Vedic diet, exercise, daily routine and seasonal routines, and physiological purification techniques; and lastly, the powerful beneficial influences of the Environment Approach that can be obtained using Vedic architecture, collective consciousness, the cycles and rhythms of nature, and Vedic sounds.

You can start your Total Heart Health program with any one of these approaches at any time. Scientific research and clinical experience have shown that all of the Vedic technologies recommended in this book are effective on their own and will contribute to your better health. However, for those who prefer a more intensive approach or faster pace, using more than one of these approaches at the same time to prevent or reverse heart disease will bring results faster and with greater efficacy. Put simply, the more you do from different angles, the more benefits you'll receive from those angles. This is an additive effect. Moreover, when Mind, Body, and Environment Approaches are used in combination, the total effect on the heart is even greater than the sum of their individual effects. This is the power of synergy. This final section presents the scientific research on the value of adopting a multifaceted approach for total heart health.

Scientific research and clinical experience with thousands of participants has demonstrated that utilizing any one of the three approaches of the Maharishi Vedic Approach to Health will bring benefits to your health and the health of your heart. Additional research and experience with patients has shown that using two or all three approaches will result in more complete benefits faster. Indeed, it is a major principle of the Maharishi Vedic Approach to Health that all three levels of influence—the mind, the body, and the environment—contribute to heart disease. Therefore, your ideal Total Heart Health program would incorporate modalities aimed at all three of these levels. Of course, you can begin with any of the approaches as your circumstances allow.

Many people who have followed the Total Heart Health program find that as they begin to experience a decrease in symptoms, they also experience more energy and vitality, and naturally want to accelerate their progress by doing more for their health. For many people, the centerpiece of their heart disease prevention and treatment program is the Transcendental Meditation technique. As you know by now, this unique form of meditation has holistic benefits not only for the mind, but also for the body and environment. Start where you are able to and add additional techniques and routines as you experience benefits and your circumstances allow. These approaches are complementary to modern medical care, but always consult your physician or healthcare provider before making any changes in your conventional medical care.

THE BENEFITS OF USING MORE THAN ONE APPROACH

One of the most persuasive studies on the increased benefit of simultaneously using multiple approaches of the Total Heart Health program was conducted recently at St. Joseph's Hospital and Health Center in Chicago, in collaboration with our team at the Institute for Natural Medicine and Prevention at Maharishi University of Management. The surprising results were published in the *American Journal of Cardiology.* In this randomized-controlled clinical trial, fifty-seven men and women over age sixty-five, who were normally healthy, were assigned to one of three groups. All groups were matched at baseline for similarity of cardiovascular risk factors.

One group followed both the Mind and Body Approaches of the Total Heart Health program. The specific techniques included the Transcendental Meditation program, Vedic diet and exercise, and the herbal antioxidant supplement *Maharishi Amrit Kalash.* The second group followed a conventional heart disease prevention program designed to provide advice that mainstream doctors in the community give their heart patients. This comparison program involved attending health-education classes, maintaining a low-fat diet, engaging in aerobic exercise, and taking a conventional multivitamin and mineral supplement. The third group continued their usual health care with their conventional doctors with no extra treatment program. All the men and women continued with their usual medical care of medications and/or other recommendations provided by their conventional physicians. Subjects were randomly assigned to their respective programs (thus avoiding self-selection bias). The participants followed their programs for one year.

Before each participant began the program, researchers measured the extent of atherosclerosis present in the carotid artery of each person using a high-resolution ultrasound technique known as *ultrasonography*. The thickness of the wall of the carotid artery in the neck has been found to be an accurate predictor of risk for future heart attack and stroke. After one year of home-based participation, forty-six of the participants returned for retesting.

What did researchers find? In the group using the Total Heart Health program's Mind and Body Approaches, there was a reduction in the thickness of the artery wall, which corresponds to a 10 percent reduction in the probability of future heart disease compared with the controls. Yet, surprisingly, those participants who were at highest risk for heart disease—that is, those who already had one or more of the conventional risk factors for heart disease (hypertension, high cholesterol, obesity, diabetes, and cigarette addiction)—exhibited a reduction in atherosclerosis, which corresponds to a 33 percent decrease on average in the risk for future heart attacks or strokes compared with the other groups. This outcome was greater than the effects reported in other studies using several cholesterol-lowering and blood-pressure-lowering medications, or with practicing the Transcendental Meditation program alone.

In addition, in the Total Heart Health program group, there was more than 80 percent compliance. In the group following the conventional medical recommendations, there was an average of 54 percent compliance. This means that most people in the Total Heart Health program group found their program easier to stick with than the dietary restrictions and exercise programs traditionally recommended for heart disease prevention. And finally, in the Total Heart Health program group, 80 percent of all subjects and 100 percent of high-risk individuals (defined above) showed a regression in atherosclerosis.

What are the implications of these findings? The results suggest that when two or more approaches of the Total Heart Health program are used together, they do indeed have a synergistic effect that stimulates the body's own self-repair and balancing mechanisms to a greater extent than is predicted by adding their individual effects. The result is a healthier cardiovascular system and more effective prevention of heart disease than is typically found with conventional medical approaches to heart disease.

A study conducted by Dr. David Orme-Johnson and colleagues at Maharishi University of Management also reinforced the idea of extra benefits from using multiple approaches of the Maharishi Vedic Approach to Health to prevent heart disease. The results were published in the *American Journal of Managed*

Care. In this research, nearly 700 normally healthy individuals who selected their own modalities from among the three approaches of the Maharishi Vedic Approach to Health were studied. Their choice of modalities included the Transcendental Meditation and TM-Sidhi programs, Vedic diet, Vedic exercise, daily and seasonal routines, herbal supplements, physiological purification procedures, and techniques from the Environment Approach.

Researchers analyzed data for these men and women, and compared their healthcare utilization patterns to those of 4,000 normally healthy control subjects matched for age, geographical location, and occupation. (Subjects in both groups were faculty and staff at Midwestern universities.) Comparisons were also made to norms determined for 600,000 subjects whose data were accumulated in an insurance company database over an eleven-year period. The researchers observed that those using multiple modalities of the Maharishi Vedic Approach to Health, on average, showed about 60 percent lower rates of medical-care utilization than the control subjects. Hospital admission rates for cardiovascular disease were more than ten times lower than for the control group. The greatest reductions were seen for participants older than age forty-five.

Two additional studies were published by Professor Tony Nader, Dr. Stuart Rothenberg, and colleagues in collaboration with the Institute for Natural Medicine and Prevention that reached a similar conclusion about the effects of combining approaches used in the Total Heart Health program. In both studies, the participants had long-standing, difficult-to-treat, chronic diseases. Each of these studies presented outcomes from a series of patients with difficult-to-treat chronic disorders. The number of cases was not large, nor were the studies randomized, controlled clinical trials, as were the earlier studies mentioned. However, the results were encouraging.

Patients in these studies participated in in-residence physiological purification programs, practiced the Transcendental Meditation and advanced TM-Sidhi programs, followed Vedic diets, exercise and daily routines, used multiple herbal preparations, learned self-pulse diagnosis, utilized Maharishi Vedic Sound therapies, and Vedic engineering procedures. After leaving the in-residence program, subjects continued with home programs of meditation, diet, exercise, and herbal supplements. Some incorporated Maharishi Vedic Architecture into their homes and continued their participation in Maharishi Vedic Astrology and Vedic engineering programs.

Using standard clinical measures for their respective disorders such as office blood-pressure measurements, blood glucose and hemoglobin A1C (for diabetes), standard tests by their neurologists for Parkinson's disease and multiple sclerosis, and others, the results showed improvements in symptoms and objective measures of advanced hypertension, diabetes, Parkinson's disease, multiple sclerosis, chronic back pain, and obesity. Many of these results were remarkable. One patient who had experienced kidney damage decades earlier was put on antihypertensive medications, and was told that she would have to be on these medications for life. However, by the end of the in-residence portion of the program, she was able to be tapered off the medications and maintain normal blood pressure.

Many inferences can be drawn from these studies. But the most important finding is the consistency and effectiveness with which those who used multiple approaches of the Total Heart Health program were able to tap into the body's own healing mechanisms, an accomplishment that resulted in disease prevention or chronic disease regression in extraordinary ways.

A VISION OF TOTAL HEART HEALTH

The Total Heart Health program with its multifaceted Mind, Body, and Environment Approaches gives you the foundation for developing and maintaining total heart health so that you can begin to live a longer, happier, more vibrant life. Because all three approaches operate at the basis of your physiology, at the level of the unified field of natural law, each technique within these categories— be it mental, physical, or environmental—will have profound effects on your entire physiology.

The Mind Approach offers the Transcendental Meditation program with its holistic benefits of reducing stress, a major contributing factor in heart disease and most illnesses, while promoting the health of both the mind and body. Physiological research has shown that practicing the Transcendental Meditation program develops orderliness of brain functioning, simultaneously lowers stress hormone levels, blood pressure, lipid levels, and smoking, and slows or reverses atherosclerosis, heart disease, and biological aging. This is all due to regularly experiencing the fourth state of consciousness, transcendental consciousness, which enlivens the body's own inner intelligence.

The Body Approach restores balance at the quantum mechanical level of your physiology as described thousands of years ago by ancient Vedic texts and confirmed by modern science. This approach uses diet, herbal and nutritional supplements, exercise, daily and seasonal routines, and physiological purification procedures. Scientific research on these techniques has shown that they elicit holistic improvements in mental and physical health, including the prevention and treatment of heart disease and its major risk factors. Modern medicine has corroborated the value of a diet high in fruits and vegetables, whole grains, and healthy fats, as recommended by the Total Heart Health program, in large studies that demonstrated less cardiovascular disease and mortality with this type of diet. Studies of Maharishi Vedic herbal preparations indicate that they are among the most powerful antioxidants known to modern science, which helps to explain their potent effects on restoring physiological balance.

The Environment Approach addresses the effects of your home and workplace, the collective consciousness around you, and the influences of cycles and rhythms of nature associated with the sun, moon, stars, and planets. Maharishi Vedic Architecture, the Maharishi Effect (on collective consciousness), Maharishi Vedic Astrology and Vedic engineering, and Maharishi Vedic Sound programs all help to strengthen the connection of the individual's physiology with the unified field of natural law that governs the structures and functions of the entire universe around us. Scientific research and extensive clinical experience with these modalities has demonstrated lower rates of heart disease and other chronic disorders in individuals living in buildings designed according to principles of healthy architecture; rapid reductions in symptoms of heart disease and others chronic conditions with the application of Vedic sound therapies; and reduced stress, warfare, and sickness in society when a small group of people reduce their own stress and radiate coherence through the field effect of consciousness.

Finally, when the three approaches of the Total Heart Health program are used together, their effects are more than additive—they are multiplied. The more you do, the more you benefit. Studies have shown major reversals of heart disease, as well as other serious chronic diseases, when the Mind, Body, and Environment Approaches are used together. This is due to the infinite organizing and healing power of your inner intelligence made accessible through these approaches. Yet, no matter whether you choose to take advantage of one, two, or all three approaches or selected modalities within these categories, you will experience major benefits. These approaches take different angles with the same end result, which is to remind your body what it is really like to operate as it was meant to, in tune with the intelligence of the universe. This is what truly prevents and reverses heart disease without harmful side effects and with only positive side benefits.

Your innate growth toward total health will be reflected in the society in which you live and in the world in which you exist. A natural byproduct of stress-free, healthy individuals is a stress-free, healthy world. This is the ultimate purpose and promise of the Maharishi Vedic Approach to Health and the Total Heart Health program: the unfoldment of the full potential of every individual and the creation of a world that is disease-free and problem-free, without suffering, a world that is healthy, harmonious, and peaceful.

Glossary

Agni. A term from Vedic physiology, agni refers to the processes of digestion and cellular metabolism. The seat of agni in the body is in the stomach and small intestine.

Ama. A term from Vedic physiology, ama is the byproduct of improper digestion. It is the sticky toxic remains of undigested food that obstructs the channels, or shrotas, in the body.

Arteriosclerosis. A chronic disease of thickening and hardening of the arteries that impairs blood circulation.

Atherosclerosis. The most common type of arteriosclerosis. The process in which deposits of fatty substances, cholesterol, cellular-waste products, calcium, and other substances build up in the inner lining of the arteries, especially in the coronary arteries, which supply blood, oxygen, and nutrients to the heart. This formation of atherosclerotic plaques in the arteries that impair the blood supply to the heart itself is the underlying disease process of coronary heart disease, also known as coronary artery disease. Atherosclerosis of the arteries in the heart is the most common cause of heart attack. Atherosclerosis in the brain is the most common cause of stroke.

Atma. A Vedic term that signifies each person's innermost self. Atma is experienced as transcendental consciousness, or the least excited state of consciousness during the practice of the Transcendental Meditation technique. In quantum physics, the description of the Unified Field of Natural Law parallels the Vedic description of Atma. According to both ancient Vedic science and modern science, this field contains the information and knowledge that directs the more manifest expressions of human physiology. In this regard, Atma is analogous to DNA, which contains the instructions, or blueprint, for the entire human body as it develops throughout the life course. Therefore, Atma is also considered the inner intelligence of the human physiology.

Cardiovascular disease. A general term encompassing diseases of the heart and cardiovascular system. Coronary heart disease, also called *coronary artery disease,* and stroke are the principal categories of cardiovascular disease. Cardiovascular disease accounts for almost half of all deaths in the United States and is the leading cause of death worldwide. Hypertension, a major risk factor for coronary heart disease and stroke, may also be considered a cardiovascular disease.

Chronobiology. The knowledge and study of the effects of time and rhythmical phenomena on physiological processes.

Chronomedicine. Branch of medicine that is concerned with the causes, diagnoses, prevention and treatments of abnormalities in our biological rhythms.

Consciousness. In the Vedic system, consciousness signifies awareness. Previously, scientists believed that there were three basic states of consciousness, or qualities of awareness: waking, dreaming, and deep sleep. During the practice of the Transcendental Meditation technique, a fourth major state of consciousness known as *transcendental consciousness* is experienced. This state is characterized by silent inner wakefulness coupled with reduced physiological activity. Thus, it has been called a state of restful alertness or the least excited state of consciousness. According to the Maharishi Vedic Approach to Health, consciousness is the source of creativity and intelligence in the human mind and body. This inner intelligence of human physiology is also the inner intelligence of all of nature (see *Atma;* Unified field, Unified field of natural law).

Coronary heart disease. Also known as coronary artery disease; the most common type of cardiovascular disease. Coronary heart disease leads to angina pectoris (chest pain), heart attacks (myocardial infarctions), cardiac arrhythmias, heart failure, and sudden cardiac death. Coronary heart disease is due to atherosclerosis of the coronary arteries.

Cosmic counterparts. Cosmic counterparts refer to the sun, moon, stars, and planets and their precise relationship to structures and functions in the human brain, cell, DNA, and all the parts of the human body. Discovery of the one-to-one relationship between the fundamental structures and functions of human physiology and the fundamental structures and functions of natural law in the cosmos was made by neuroscientist Professor Tony Nader, M.D., Ph.D.

Dhatus. A term from Vedic physiology, dhatus refers to the tissues of the body. The seven dhatus are formed in sequence starting with rasa (the plasma component of blood) and ending with sukra (reproductive tissue).

Doshas. A term from Vedic physiology that refers to the three physiological principles or operators governing all the processes and activities in the body. The doshas have functions in all of nature as well as in the human body.

Heart disease. A type of cardiovascular disease. In this book, heart disease refers to coronary heart disease caused by atherosclerosis. This disease process is the basis of most heart attacks (and many strokes). Heart disease is the number-one cause of death and serious disability in the United States.

Inner intelligence of the body. The source of creativity and intelligence of natural law in the human physiology. In physics, this is called the unified field of natural law. In physiological terms, this inner intelligence is embodied in the DNA, the underlying basis of the physical structure and function of the body.

Kapha dosha. One of the three governing principles of the physiology. Kapha dosha is responsible for and regulates bodily structure, including building tissues, and the amount of water and fat in the cells and tissues.

Laws of nature. The laws that govern the structure and function of the universe and everything contained within it. These include the laws of all fields of science, including physics, mathematics, chemistry, physiology, ecology, astronomy, cosmology, and others. Scientific knowledge about the laws of nature governing biochemical and physiological processes provides the theoretical basis for all the applied methods, approaches, and technologies in the field of medicine.

Maharishi Gandharva Veda. Part of the Maharishi Vedic Approach to Health, a type of sound therapy based on the music and rhythms of nature. According to the discovery of Professor Tony Nader, M.D., Ph.D., Gandharva Veda music correlates with the rhythms and cycles of the heart.

Maharishi Vedic Astrology, or Maharishi Jyotish. One of the forty aspects of Veda and Vedic literature and part of the Maharishi Vedic Approach to Health. This branch includes knowledge about the cycles and rhythms of nature that may be used to calculate future health trends. It includes knowledge of technologies to optimize these trends (see Maharishi Yagya). This field is analogous to chronobiology and chronomedicine in modern medicine.

Maharishi Vedic Architecture, or Maharishi Sthapatya Veda. One of the forty aspects of Veda and Vedic literature and part of the Maharishi Vedic Approach to Health. This is a scientific system of healthy architecture from the ancient Vedic tradition that incorporates principles of direction, placement, and proportion to create healthy buildings for homes, schools, and communities.

Maharishi Yagya. Closely interrelated with Maharishi Vedic Astrology. This technology of the Maharishi Vedic Approach to Health is used to prevent unwanted environmental influences from having a negative impact on life and well-being. Also known as *Vedic engineering,* the Maharishi Yagya program not only counteracts unwanted influences that were generated in the past, but also enhances positive trends in health and life in general.

Ojas. The refined and nourishing byproduct of digestion that strengthens the body and makes it resilient to disease and aging.

Pitta dosha. One of the three governing principles of the physiology. Pitta dosha regulates and is responsible for digestion, metabolism, energy production, and heat, among other functions in the body.

Shrotas. The innumerable channels of communication and transportation through-out the body. Shrotas carry nutrients and waste products in and out of cells, tis-sues, and organs of the body. They can be visible to the human eye, such as the coronary arteries, veins, tear ducts, and the ear canals, or microscopic such as a pore in a cell membrane. If the shrotas become disrupted or blocked, physiolog-ical processes are hindered and disease may result. Heart disease is an example of a disease of blocked shrotas.

Transcendental consciousness. One of the four major states of consciousness. A unique state of restful alertness distinct from waking, dreaming, and deep sleep that is characterized by enhanced integration of brain functioning and deep phys-iological rest. The Transcendental Meditation technique is a systematic and easy method to experience transcendental consciousness and gain its benefits for health. In Vedic terms, this state is also called Atma, or the direct experience of the unified field of natural law (see next entry).

Unified field, unified field of natural law. A groundbreaking discovery that began with the work of Albert Einstein and continues to be refined in the twenti-eth and twenty-first centuries by quantum field theorists in quantum mechanics. The most recent elaboration is called the "string theory." These theories at the cutting edge of modern physics describe a single underlying, unmanifest field of natural law from which all forms and phenomena in the universe sequentially emerge. This is the field of nature's intelligence, a field of total knowledge. In Vedic terms, this is identified as the inner intelligence of the mind and body, or Atma.

Vata dosha. One of the three governing principles of the physiology. Vata dosha leads the movements of all the other doshas. Vata dosha regulates movement in every part of the body, including heartbeat; the movement of blood through the tissues; the exchange of air, food, and water in each cell; and the transmission of nerve impulses and signals that urge cells to operate.

Veda. A Vedic term that means knowledge. Traditionally, held to be the total knowledge of life. The Veda and its associated Vedic literature have been trans-mitted in oral tradition for thousands of years. In recent times, the Veda and Vedic literature have been recorded in sets of books. Much of the original meaning and value of this knowledge is said to have been lost in the last centuries. In the past fifty years, Maharishi Mahesh Yogi has revived and systematized the original knowledge of Veda and Vedic literature in the light of modern science and empirical research. Maharishi has explained that Veda is the unified field of natural law. As such, it was uncreated by man and is eternal. The fluctuations, or sounds of the Veda, are said to be indicative of the fluctuations, or sounds, of natural law emerging from the unified field. Maharishi describes the human body and mind as the embodiment of Veda and a living replica of natural law. The relationship of the human body to Veda was confirmed by the discoveries of neuroscientist Professor Tony Nader, M.D., Ph.D.

Vedic. Refers to the Veda. The Vedic tradition is the world's oldest system of health care and total knowledge. It has been transmitted in oral form by the Vedic families of India for thousands of years. It has been recently revived and restored to completeness in a scientific framework by Maharishi Mahesh Yogi.

Vedic literature. The most fundamental aspect of the Veda and Vedic literature (see Veda) is the first discipline, called Rik Veda. Rik Veda is said to represent the holistic value of the dynamics of natural law. The other thirty-nine aspects of Veda and Vedic literature assume one predominant quality of natural law as its specialty. For example, the Yoga branch of Vedic literature has the theme of unifying, oneness of all things. In this book, we refer to the first four aspects of the Veda and Vedic literature, Rik, Sama, Yajur, and Atharva Veda, as "Veda" and to the other thirty-six branches collectively as the "Vedic literature."

Resources

For more information on the Total Heart Health program,
visit **www.totalhearthealth.info**.

SERVICES AND PRODUCTS

Many of the products you may want to use in your Total Heart Health program
can be obtained at your local health food store or other natural products shops.
However, some products and services need to be obtained from the specialized
sources listed in this section. While every effort has been made to include the
most up-to-date information at the time of publication, addresses, telephone
numbers, e-mail addresses, and website links may change.

MAHARISHI VEDIC HEALTH CARE

Maharishi Vedic Health programs are prevention-oriented, time-tested, free
from harmful side effects, and easily applied. The Maharishi Vedic Approach to
Health enlivens consciousness at the basis of one's physiology to restore and
maintain health and to promote higher states of well-being and enlightenment.
To locate a physician or consultant trained in the Maharishi Vedic Approach to
Health in your area, contact your local Maharishi Peace Palace or Maharishi Enlightenment Center (see page 232) or one of the following health facilities:

The Raj Ayurveda Health Spa
A world-class health spa offering luxurious and powerful purification treatments
to help remove the damaging effects of stress, fatigue, impurities and environ-
mental toxins, thereby stimulating the body's natural rejuvenating abilities.
　　Address: 1734 Jasmine Avenue
　　Maharishi Vedic City, IA 52556
　　Phone: 1-800-248-9050 or 641-472-9580
　　Fax: (641) 472-2496
　　E-mail: theraj@lisco.com
　　Website: www.theraj.com

Maharishi Vedic Health Center

A leading medical spa for individuals with chronic disorders, also offering natural, noninvasive programs for prevention of disease, rejuvenation, and the promotion of ideal health.

> Address: 679 George Hill Road
> Lancaster, MA 01523
> Phone: (877) 890-8600 or (508) 365-4549
> Fax: (978) 368-7557
> E-mail: info@lancasterhealth.com
> Website: www.lancasterhealth.com/splash.html

Maharishi Vedic Vibration Technology (MVVT)

Maharishi Vedic Vibration Technology has brought relief to thousands suffering from chronic disorders, including people with arthritis, asthma, anxiety, back pain, depression, digestive problems, headache, and insomnia.

> Phone: (800) 431-9680
> E-mail: applications@vedicvibration.com
> Website: vedicvibration.com

MAHARISHI VEDIC ARCHITECTURE

Maharishi Vedic Architecture uses ancient Vedic design principles to guide the building of homes, offices, and communities that are in accord with natural law. This creates good health, happiness, and good fortune for the people who inhabit these buildings. For consulting services in the United States, contact your local Maharishi Peace Palace or Enlightenment Center:

> Phone: (888) LEARN TM (1-888-532-7686)
> Website: vedicarchitecture.org

For countries outside of the United States, Canada and the Caribbean, contact:

> International Institute of Maharishi Sthapatya Veda
> Maharishi Vedic University
> E-mail: VedicArchitecture@Maharishi.Net
> Website: www.sthapatyaveda.com

MAHARISHI VEDIC ASTROLOGY AND MAHARISHI YAGYA PROGRAMS

To find out more about Maharishi Vedic Astrology (Jyotish) consultations and Maharishi Yagya performances, contact one of the following Maharishi Yagya regional offices:

East Coast
    Address: P.O. Box 2213
    Kensington, MD 20891
    Tel: (301) 230-0923
    Fax: (240) 290-0418
    E-mail: MaharishiYagyaTZ9@Maharishi.net

Midwest
    Address: P.O. Box 11726
    Lexington, KY 40577
    Tel: (859) 977-0875
    Fax: (859) 977-0876
    E-mail: MaharishiYagyaTZ10@Maharishi.net

West Coast
    Address: P.O. Box 665
    Palo Alto, CA 94302
    Tel: (650) 843-0830
    Fax: (650) 843-0823
    E-mail: MaharishiYagyaTZ11@Maharishi.net

MAHARISHI VEDIC MUSIC

Maharishi Gandharva Veda music mirrors the fundamental frequencies and rhythms of nature. It is a powerful tool for dissolving tensions in the individual and the environment, creating greater integration of body and mind. To learn more:
    E-mail: mtc@ayurveda.nl
    Websites: www.maharishi-gandharva.com
                www.mumpress.com/catalog.html#music
                www.mapi.com
                www.maharishi.org/gandharva/music_selections.html
                (for a taste of Gandharva Veda music)

MAHARISHI VEDIC ORGANIC AGRICULTURE

Maharishi Vedic Organic Agriculture uses Vedic technologies to enliven the intelligence and vitality of natural law in plants, creating improved health for the farmer, the family, the nation, and the environment.

Maharishi Vedic Organic Agriculture Institute

This institute provides Maharishi Vedic Organic Agriculture certification for food that is not only free from harmful chemical residues and genetic modification, but also is lively in the full intelligence of natural law.

Address: 1431 South Pennsylvania Ave., Suite #3
Casper, WY 82609
Phone: (307) 237-1055
Fax: (307) 237-5547
E-mail: MVOAI@Maharishi.net
Website: mvoai.org

Maharishi Ayurveda Products International (MAPI)

Manufacturer and distributor of the world's foremost herbal formulas based on the traditional Vedic texts. MAPI is an excellent source of products mentioned in this book, including herbal supplements, teas, oils, music, books, and tapes, and provides detailed product information.

Address: 1068 Elkton Drive
Colorado Springs, CO 80907
Phone: (800) 255-8332 or (719) 260-5500
Fax: (719) 260-7400
E-mail: questions@mapi.com
Website: mapi.com

EDUCATIONAL RESOURCES

MAHARISHI PEACE PALACES AND MAHARISHI ENLIGHTENMENT CENTERS

At Maharishi Peace Palaces, you'll find programs to rejuvenate your mind and body, address chronic disorders, and develop higher states of consciousness. All of the consciousness-based technologies and programs have their origins in the ancient Vedic civilization of India. They have been scientifically validated by leading research institutions and taught by experts with decades of personal experience. Even the distinctive natural architecture of the Maharishi Peace Palace enhances refined states of consciousness and inner peace. To locate the Maharishi Peace Palace or Maharishi Enlightenment Center closest to you, use the following contact information:

Phone: (888) LEARN TM (1-888-532-7686)
Website: www.maharishipeacepalace.org or www.tm.org

Transcendental Meditation Program
The Transcendental Meditation program of Maharishi Mahesh Yogi is the single most effective meditation technique available for gaining deep relaxation, eliminating stress, promoting health, increasing creativity and intelligence, and attaining inner happiness and fulfillment. Courses are offered through local Maharishi Peace Palaces and Maharishi Enlightenment Centers.

> Phone: (888) LEARN TM (1-888-532-7686)
>
> Website: www.tm.org

TM-Sidhi Program
The TM-Sidhi program is an advanced program of the Maharishi Vedic Approach to Health that develops mind-body coordination. The TM-Sidhi program is a natural extension of the Transcendental Meditation program and may be learned after two months of regular practice of the Transcendental Meditation technique. Practice of the TM-Sidhi program accelerates the progress of the individual toward realizing his full potential for total health—the state of enlightenment. Courses are offered through local Maharishi Peace Palaces and Maharishi Enlightenment Centers.

> Phone: (888) LEARN TM (1-888-532-7686)
>
> Websites: www.tm.org or www.tm.org/sidhi

SCHOOLS AND UNIVERSITIES

The following Consciousness-Based educational programs, universities and schools enliven the total potential of brain physiology in students, systematically unfolding inner intelligence, health, happiness and creativity. Using scientifically proven technologies such as the Transcendental Meditation technique, students grow in the ability to achieve anything, as they enliven the unlimited creative potential in their own consciousness.

Maharishi Open University (MOU)
Courses that you can take at home via satellite and Internet links awaken the participant's inner intelligence through the unique combination of knowledge and experience of the total potential of natural law.

> Phone: (800) 765-5421
>
> Website: www.mou.org

Maharishi University of Management (MUM)

This unique university's consciousness-based approach develops higher states of consciousness while offering degree and nondegree programs in a wide range of arts and sciences at both the undergraduate and graduate levels.

Address: 1000 North Fourth Street
Fairfield, IA 52557
Phone: (800) 369-6480 or (641) 472-1110
Fax: (641) 472-1179
Website: admissions@mum.edu

Maharishi School of the Age of Enlightenment

Consciousness-based education for preschool to grade 12. Located on the campus of Maharishi University of Management.

Address: Business Office
804 North Third Street
Fairfield, IA 52556
Phone: (866) 472-MSAE (6723) or (641) 472-9400
Fax: (641) 472-1211
E-mail: info@msae.edu
Website: www.maharishischooliowa.org

Consciousness-Based Education Association (CBE)

Offers scientifically validated Consciousness-Based educational programs to schools, colleges, and universities throughout the world. More than forty years of experience have shown that these programs improve educational outcomes, reduce stress and antisocial behavior, increase creativity and intelligence, and unfold the inner happiness of students and teachers of all cultural and educational backgrounds.

Address: National Office
Consciousness-Based Education Association
1100 University Manor Drive, B-24
Fairfield, IA 52556
Phone: (800) 472-8285
website: www.cbeprograms.org
E-mail: info@CBEprograms.org

Vedic Communities

This is an entire city designed according to Maharishi Vedic Architecture to promote health, happiness, and good fortune. Through holistic health care, organic agriculture, and consciousness-based educational programs that focus on developing the full potential of the student, the city is applying Vedic knowledge to promote health, happiness, and a higher quality of life.

Address: City Hall
1973 Grand Drive
Maharishi Vedic City, IA 52556
Phone: (641) 470-7000
Fax: (641) 470-7001
E-mail: Information@maharishivediccity.net
Website: maharishivediccity.net

HEALTH EDUCATION: SHORT COURSES

The following short courses are available through your local Maharishi Peace Palace or Maharishi Enlightenment Center.

Good Health Through Prevention: This sixteen-hour course includes specific recommendations to help prevent ill health using daily and seasonal routines, individualized diet, other health-promoting behaviors, and development of higher states of consciousness.

Self-Pulse Reading for Prevention: This introductory course provides the theory and practical technique for detecting balance and imbalance in the body through self-pulse reading. The course also describes measures to correct imbalances before disease arises.

Diet, Digestion, and Nutrition: This course provides profound principles and practical knowledge of how to promote good health through proper diet, digestion, and nutrition. Participants learn to select their diet based on the state of their physiology and the season and to promote optimal nourishment and health through balanced digestion.

The Maharishi Yoga Program: This course gives a comprehensive understanding of the nature and attainment of Yoga, which is the unification of individual and cosmic life. Participants are trained in Maharishi Yoga program postures and breathing exercises, which promote mind-body integration and support balanced good health.

BOOKS

These and other excellent resource books are available from Maharishi University of Management Press, Maharishi Ayurveda Products International, or your local bookseller.

Maharishi University of Management Press
Address: DB 1155
Fairfield, IA 52557-1155
Phone: (800) 831-6523
Website: www.mumpress.com

Maharishi Ayurveda Products International
Address: 1068 Elkton Drive
Colorado Springs, CO 80907
Phone: (800) 255-8332 or (719) 260-5500
Fax: (719) 260-7400
E-mail: questions@mapi.com
Website: mapi.com

Human Physiology: Expression of Veda and the Vedic Literature, 4th Edition, by Professor Tony Nader, M.D., Ph.D. (Maharishi Vedic University, 2001). This groundbreaking work details the relationship between the forty branches of Veda and the Vedic literature and their corresponding parts in the human physiology.

The Science of Being and Art of Living, Reissue Edition, by Maharishi Mahesh Yogi (Plume, 2001). The summation of both the practical wisdom of integrated life advanced by the Vedic scientists of ancient India and the growth of scientific thinking in the present-day Western world. It presents a philosophy of life in fulfillment, and brings forth a practice suitable for all people to glorify all aspects of their day-to-day life.

Maharishi Mahesh Yogi on the Bhagavad-Gita: A New Translation and Commentary, Chapters 1–6, Reprint Edition, by Maharishi Mahesh Yogi (Penguin, 1990). Maharishi calls the *Bhagavad-Gita,* "the essence of Vedic Literature and a complete guide to practical life." It provides "all that is needed to raise the consciousness of man to the highest possible level." Maharishi reveals the deep, universal truths of life that speak to the needs and aspirations of everyone.

Maharishi's Forum of Natural Law and National Law for Doctors: Perfect Health for Everyone—Disease-Free Society, by Maharishi Mahesh Yogi (Maharishi Vedic University Press, 1995). This book introduces a prevention-oriented, comprehensive, natural law-based, all-enriching system of perfect health. The centuries old medicine-predominated approach to health has failed to eliminate sickness and suffering. This is because medicine alone is too superficial to influence all the innumerable values that constitute the structure of life and its evolution. Only a holistic approach that takes into consideration all aspects of mind and body together can be successful in handling health.

References

Introduction

Chalmers RA, Clements G, Schenkluhn H, Weinless M, eds. *Scientific Research on Maharishi's Transcendental Meditation and TM-Sidhi Program: Collected Papers,* vols. 2–4. Vlodrop, The Netherlands: MVU Press, 1989.

Eisenberg DM, Davis RB, Ettner SL, et al. "Trends in alternative medicine use in the United States, 1990-1997: results of a follow-up national survey." *Journal of the American Medical Association* 1998; 280:1569–1575.

Hagelin JS. "Is consciousness the unified field? A field theorist's perspective." *Modern Science and Vedic Science* 1987; 1:28–87.

Hagelin JS. "Restructuring physics from it foundation in light of Maharishi's Vedic Science." *Modern Science and Vedic Science* 1989; 3: 3–72.

Maharishi Mahesh Yogi. *The Science of Being and Art of Living.* New York, NY: Plume/Penguin Putnam, 2001.

Nader T. *Human Physiology—Expression of Veda and the Vedic Literature.* Vlodrop, The Netherlands: MVU Press, 2000.

Orme-Johnson DW, Farrow JT. *Scientific Research on the Transcendental Meditation Program: Collected Papers,* Vol 1. Seelisberg, Switzerland: Maharishi European Research University MIU Press, 1977.

Starfield, B. "Is U.S. health really the best in the world?" *Journal of the American Medical Association* 2000; 284: 483–485.

Wallace RK, Orme-Johnson DW, Dillbeck MC, eds. *Scientific Research on Maharishi's Transcendental Meditation Program: Collected Papers,* Vol 5. Fairfield, IA: MIU Press, 1993.

Chapter 1

American Heart Association. *Heart Disease and Stroke Statistics—2006 Update.* Dallas, TX: www.americanheart.org (Jan 2006).

Crawford M, Dimarco JP, Paulus W, eds. *Cardiology*. Edinburgh: C.V. Mosby, 2004.

Hoffman C, Rice D, Sung H. "Persons with chronic conditions: Their prevalence and costs." *Journal of the American Medical Association* 1996; 276:1473–1479.

Klein S, Burke LE, Bray GA, et al. "Clinical implications of obesity with specific focus on cardiovascular disease: a statement for professionals from the American Heart Association Council on Nutrition, Physical Activity, and Metabolism and endorsed by the American College of Cardiology Foundation." *Circulation* 2004; 110: 2952–2967.

Libby P. "The forgotten majority: unfinished business in cardiovascular risk reduction." *Journal of the American College of Cardiology* 2005; 46: 1225–1228.

National Institutes of Health. *Anxiety Disorders*. Publication No. 02-3879.

National Institutes of Health. *Depression*. Publication No. 02-3561, 2002.

Wang Y and Wang QJ. "The prevalence of prehypertension and hypertension among U.S. adults according to the new joint national committee guidelines: new challenges of the old problem." *Archives of Internal Medicine* 2004; 164: 2126–2134.

Zieske A, Gray M, Strong J. "Natural history and risk factors of atherosclerosis in children and youth: the PDAY study." *Pediatric Pathology and Molecular Medicine*, 2002; 21: 213–237.

Chapter 2

Baik I, Ascherio A, Rimm EB, et al. "Adiposity and mortality in men." *American Journal of Epidemiology* 2000; 152: 264–271.

Bairey Merz CN, Dwyer J, Nordstrom C, Walton KG, Salerno JW, Schneider RH. "Psychosocial stress and cardiovascular disease, part I: pathophysiological links." *Behavioral Medicine* 2002; 27: 141-146.

Brook RD, Franklin B, Cascio W, et al. Expert Panel on Population and Prevention Science of the American Heart Association. "Air pollution and cardiovascular disease: a statement for healthcare professionals from the Expert Panel on Population and Prevention Science of the American Heart Association." *Circulation* 2004; 109: 2655–2671

Eyre H, Kahn R, Robertson RM, et al. "Preventing cancer, cardiovascular disease, and diabetes: a common agenda for the American Cancer Society, the American Diabetes Association, and the American Heart Association." *Circulation* 2004; 109: 3244–3255.

Friedman M and Rosenman RH. "Emotions in cardiovascular disease." *Heart Bulletin* 1964; 13: 21–23.

Futterman LG, Lemberg L. "Anger and acute coronary events." *American Journal of Critical Care* 2002; 11: 574–576.

Kannel WB, Castelli WP, Gordon T, et al. "Serum cholesterol, lipoproteins and the risk of coronary heart disease; the Framingham Study." *Annals of Internal Medicine* 1971; 74:1–12.

Kannel WB, Dawber TR, Kagan A, et al. "Factors of risk in the development of coronary heart disease–six year follow up experience; the Framingham Study." *Annals of Internal Medicine* 1961; 55: 33–50.

Klein S, Burke LE, Bray GA, et al."Clinical implications of obesity with specific focus on cardiovascular disease: a statement for professionals from the American Heart Association Council on Nutrition, Physical Activity, and Metabolism. Endorsed by the American College of Cardiology Foundation. *Circulation* 2004; 110: 2952–2967.

Manson JE, Hsia J, Johnson KC, et al. "Estrogen plus progestin and the risk of coronary heart disease." *New England Journal of Medicine,* 2003; 349: 523–534.

Mosca L, Appel LJ, Benjamin EJ, et al. "Evidence-based guidelines for cardiovascular disease prevention in women." *Circulation* 2004; 109: 672–693.

Myers GL, Rifai N, Tracy RP, et al. and the CDC and AHA. "CDC/AHA workshop on markers of inflammation and cardiovascular disease: application to clinical and public health practice: report from the laboratory science discussion group. *Circulation* 2004; 110: e545–e549.

Pearson TA, Blair SN, Daniels SR, et al. "AHA guidelines for primary prevention of cardiovascular disease and stroke: 2002 update: consensus panel guide to comprehensive risk reduction for adult patients without coronary or other atherosclerotic vascular diseases." *Circulation* 2002; 106: 388–391.

Pope CA, Burnett RT, Thurston GD, et al. "Cardiovascular mortality and long-term exposure to particulate air pollution: epidemiological evidence of general pathophysiological pathways of disease." *Circulation* 2004; 109: 71–77.

Reed D, McGee D, Cohen J, et al. "Acculturation and coronary heart disease among Japanese men in Hawaii." *American Journal of Epidemiology* 1982; 115: 894–905.

Ridker PM, Rifai N, Rose L, et al. "Comparison of C-reactive protein and low-density lipoprotein cholesterol levels in the prediction of first cardiovascular events." *New England Journal of Medicine* 2002; 347: 1557–1565.

Rozanski A, Blumenthal JA, Kaplan J. "Impact of psychological factors on the pathogenesis of cardiovascular disease and implications for therapy." *Circulation* 1999; 99: 2192–2217.

Rozanski A, Blumenthal JA, Davidson K, et al. "The epidemiology, pathophysiology, and management of psychosocial risk factors in cardiac practice." *Journal of the American College of Cardiology* 2005; 45: 637–651.

Smith SC Jr., Blair SN, Bonow RO, et al. "AHA/ACC guidelines for preventing heart attack and death in patients with atherosclerotic cardiovascular disease, 2001 update: a statement for healthcare professionals from the American Heart Association and the American College of Cardiology." *Journal of the American College of Cardiology* 2001; 38: 1581–1583.

Smith SC Jr, Greenland P, Grundy SM. AHA Conference Proceedings. Prevention conference V: "Beyond secondary prevention—identifying the high-risk patient for primary prevention: executive summary." *Circulation* 2000; 101: 111–116.

Chapter 3

2006 Physicians Desk Reference, 60th edition. Montvale, NJ: Thomson PDR; Package Edition, November, 2005.

Barrett-Connor E, Grady D, Stefanick ML. "The rise and fall of menopausal hormone therapy." *Annual Review of Public Health* 2005; 26: 115–140.

Collins R, Peto R, MacMahon S, et al. "Blood pressure, stroke and coronary heart disease, part II. Short-term reduction in blood pressure: overview of randomized drug trials in their epidemiological context." *Lancet* 1990; 335: 827–838.

Eisenberg D, et al. "Trends in alternative medicine use in the United States, 1990-1997: results of a follow-up national survey." *Journal of the American Medical Association* 1998; 280: 1569–1575.

Freedman JE, Becker RC, Adams JE, et al. "Medication errors in acute cardiac care: an American Heart Association scientific statement from the council on clinical cardiology subcommittee on acute cardiac care, council on cardiopulmonary and critical care, council on cardiovascular nursing, and council on stroke." *Circulation* 2002; 106: 2623–2629.

Herrington DM, Reboussin DM, Brosnihan KB, et al. "Effects of estrogen replacement on the progression of coronary artery atherosclerosis." *New England Journal of Medicine* 2000; 343: 522–529.

Hulley S, Grady D, Bush T, et al. for the Heart and Estrogen/progestin Replacement Study (HERS) Research Group. "Randomized trial of estrogen plus progestin for secondary prevention of coronary heart disease in postmenopausal women." *Journal of the American Medical Association* 1998; 280: 605–613.

Kasper DL, Braunwald E, Fauci A, et al. (eds.) *Harrison's Principles of Internal Medicine,* 16th edition. New York, NY: McGraw Hill, 2004.

Mukherjee D, Nissen SE, Topol EJ. "Risk of cardiovascular events associated with selective COX-2 inhibitors." *Journal of the American Medical Association* 2001; 286: 954–959.

Pahor M, Psaty BM, Alderman MH, et al. "Health outcomes associated with calcium antagonists compared with other first-line antihypertensive therapies: a meta-analysis of randomized controlled trials." *Lancet* 2000; 356: 1949.

Psaty BM, Heckbert SR, Loepsell TD, et al. "The risk of myocardial infarction associated with antihypertensive drug therapies." *Journal of the American Medical Association* 1995; 274: 620–625.

Starfield, B. "Is U.S. health really the best in the world?" *Journal of the American Medical Association* 2000; 284: 483–485.

Versaci F, Gaspardone A, Tomai F, et al. "A comparison of coronary artery stenting with angioplasty for isolated stenosis of the proximal left anterior descending coronary artery." *The New England Journal of Medicine* 1997; 336: 817–822.

Chapter 4

Chalmers RA, Clements G, Schenkluhn H, et al., eds. *Scientific Research on Maharishi's Transcendental Meditation and TM-Sidhi Program: Collected Papers*, Vols 2–4. Vlodrop, The Netherlands: MVU Press, 1989.

Greene, Brian. *The Elegant Universe: Superstrings, Hidden Dimensions, and the Quest for the Ultimate Theory*, New York, NY: Norton, 2003.

Hagelin, JS. "Is consciousness the unified field? A field theorist's perspective." *Modern Science and Vedic Science* 1987; 1: 28–87.

Hagelin, JS. "Restructuring physics from its foundation in light of Maharishi's Vedic Science." *Modern Science and Vedic Science* 1989; 3: 3–72.

Nader, T. *Human Physiology: Expression of Veda and the Vedic Literature*. Vlodrop, The Netherlands: MVU Press, 2000.

Orme-Johnson DW, Farrow JT. *Scientific Research on the Transcendental Meditation Program: Collected Papers*, Vol 1. Seelisberg, Switzerland: Maharishi European Research University MIU Press, 1977.

Wallace RK, Orme-Johnson DW, Dillbeck MC, eds. *Scientific Research on Maharishi's Transcendental Meditation Program: Collected Papers*, Vol 5. Fairfield, IA: MUM Press, 1993.

Chapter 5

Alexander CN, Langer EJ, Newman RI, , et al. "Transcendental Meditation, mindfulness, and longevity: An experimental study with the elderly." *Journal of Personality and Social Psychology* 1989; 57: 950–964.

Alexander CN, Robinson DK, Orme-Johnson DW, Schneider RH, et al. "The effect of Transcendental Meditation compared to other methods of relaxation and meditation in reducing risk factors, morbidity, and mortality." *Homeostasis* 1994; 35: 243–264.

Alexander CN, Robinson P, Rainforth MV. "Treating and preventing alcohol, nicotine, and drug abuse through Transcendental Meditation: a review and statistical meta-analysis." *Alcoholism Treatment Quarterly* 1994; 11:13–87.

Alexander CN, Schneider RH, Clayborne M, et al. "A randomized controlled trial of stress reduction for hypertension in older African Americans." *Hypertension* 1996; 28: 228–237.

Badawi K, Wallace RK, Orme-Johnson D, et al. "Electrophysiological characteristics of respiratory suspension periods occurring during the practice of the Transcendental Mediation program." *Psychosomatic Medicine* 1984; 46: 267–276.

Bairey Merz CN, Dwyer J, Nordstrom C, Walton KG, Salerno JW, Schneider RH. "Psychosocial stress and cardiovascular disease, part I: pathophysiological links." *Behavioral Medicine,* 2002; 27: 141–146.

Barnes VA, Davis HC, Murzynowski JB, et al. "Impact of meditation on resting and ambulatory blood pressure and heart rate in youth." *Psychosomatic Medicine* 2004; 66: 909–914.

Bujatti M, Riederer P. "Serotonin, noradrenaline, dopamine metabolites in Transcendental Meditation technique." *Journal of Neural Transmission* 1976; 39: 257– 267.

Castillo-Richmond A, Schneider R, Alexander C, et al. "Effects of stress reduction on carotid atherosclerosis in hypertensive African Americans." *Stroke* 2000; 31:5 568–573.

Cooper MJ, Aygen MM. "Effect of Transcendental Meditation on serum cholesterol and blood pressure." *Harefuah: The Journal of the Israeli Medical Association* 1978; 95: 1–2.

Cooper MJ, Aygen MM. "Transcendental Meditation in the management of hypercholesterolemia." *Journal of Human Stress* 1979; 5: 24–27.

Dillbeck MC, Orme-Johnson DW. "Physiological differences between Transcendental Meditation and rest." *American Psychologist* 1987; 42: 879–881.

Eppley KR, Abrams A, Shear J. "Differential effects of relaxation techniques on trait anxiety: a meta-analysis." *Journal of Clinical Psychology* 1989; 45: 957–974.

Fields JZ, Walton KG, Schneider RH, et al. "Effect of a multimodality natural medicine program on carotid atherosclerosis in older subjects: a pilot trial of Maharishi Vedic Medicine." *American Journal of Cardiology* 2002; 89: 952–958.

Gelderloos P, Walton KG, Orme-Johnson DW, et al. "Effectiveness of the Transcendental Meditation program in preventing and treating substance misuse: a review." *International Journal of the Addictions* 1991; 26: 293–325.

Herron RE, Hillis SL, Mandarino JV, et al. "The impact of the Transcendental Meditation program on government payments to physicians in Quebec." *American Journal of Health Promotion* 1996; 10: 208–216.

Infante JR, Torres-Avisbal M, Pinel P, et al. "Catecholamine levels in practitioners of the Transcendental Meditation technique." *Physiology and Behavior* 2001; 72: 141–146.

Jevning R, Wilson AF, Davidson JM. "Adrenocortical activity during mediation." *Hormones and Behavior* 1978; 10: 54–60.

Jevning R, Wallace RK, Biedebach M. "The physiology of meditation: a review. A wakeful hypometabolic integrated response." *Neuroscience and Biobehavioral Reviews* 1992: 16: 415–424.

MacLean CR, Walton KG, Wenneberg SR, Levitsky DK, Mandarino JP, Waziri R, Hillis SL, Schneider RH. "Effects of the Transcendental Meditation program on adaptive mechanisms: changes in hormone levels and responses to stress after 4 months of practice." *Psychoneuroendocrinology* 1997; 22: 277–295.

McEwen, B. *The End of Stress as We Know It.* Washington, DC: Joseph Henry Press, 2002.

Orme-Johnson DW. "Medical care utilization and the Transcendental Meditation program." *Psychosomatic Medicine* 1987; 49: 493–507.

Mills PJ, Schneider RH, Hill D, et al. "Beta-adrenergic receptor sensitivity in subjects practicing Transcendental Meditation." *Journal of Psychosomatic Research* 1990; 34: 29–33.

Orme-Johnson DW, Walton KG. "All approaches to preventing and reversing the effects of stress are not the same." *American Journal of Health Promotion* 1998; 12: 297–299.

Orme-Johnson DW. "Medical care utilization and the Transcendental Meditation program." *Psychosomatic Medicine* 1987; 49: 493–507.

Schneider RH, Nidich SI, Salerno JW, et al. "Lower lipid peroxide levels in practitioners of the Transcendental Meditation program." *Psychosom Med.* 1998; 60: 38–41.

Schneider RH, Staggers F, Alexander C, et al. "A randomized controlled trial of stress reduction in African Americans treated for hypertension for over one year." *American Journal of Hypertension* 2005; 18: 88–98.

Schneider RH, Staggers F, Alexander C, et al. "A randomized controlled trial of stress reduction of hypertension in older African Americans." *Hypertension* 1995; 26: 820–827.

Schneider RH, Alexander CN, Staggers F, et al. "Long-term effects of stress reduction on mortality in persons > 55 years of age with systemic hypertension." *American Journal of Cardiology* 2005; 95: 1060–1064.

Schneider RH, Cavanaugh W, Boncheff S. "Cost Reductions Through Better Health." *Business and Health,* 1986; Nov: 39–42.

Wallace, Robert Keith. *The Physiology of Consciousness.* Fairfield IA: Maharishi International University Press, 1995.

Wallace RK, Benson H. "The physiology of meditation." *Scientific American* 1972; 226: 84–90.

Wallace RK, Benson H, Wilson AF. "A wakeful hypometabolic physiologic state." *American Journal of Physiology* 1971; 221: 795–799.

Wallace RK, Silver J, Mills PJ, et al. "Systolic blood pressure and long-term practice of the Transcendental Meditation and TM-Sidhi program: effects of TM on systolic blood pressure." *Psychosomatic Medicine* 1983; 45: 41–46.

Walton KG, Schneider RH, Nidich SI. "Review of controlled research on the Transcendental Meditation program and cardiovascular disease: risk factors, morbidity and mortality." *Cardiology in Review* 2004; 12(5): 262–266.

Walton KG, Schneider RH, Nidich SI, et al. "Psychosocial stress and cardiovascular disease 3: Practicality and policy implications of the Transcendental Meditation program." *Behavioral Medicine* 2005; 30: 173–183.

Walton KG, Schneider RH, Nidich SI, et al. "Psychosocial stress and cardiovascular disease 2: effectiveness of the Transcendental Meditation program in treatment and prevention." *Behavioral Medicine* 2002; 28:106-123.

Zamarra JW, Schneider RH, Besseghini I, et al. "Usefulness of the Transcendental Meditation program in the treatment of patients with coronary artery disease." *American Journal of Cardiology* 1996; 78: 77–80.

Chapter 6

Alexander CN, Robinson DK, Orme-Johnson DW, Schneider RH, et al. "The effect of Transcendental Meditation compared to other methods of relaxation and meditation in reducing risk factors, morbidity, and mortality." *Homeostasis* 1994; 35: 243–264.

Dillbeck MC, Orme-Johnson DW. "Physiological differences between Transcendental Meditation and rest." *American Psychologist* 1987; 42: 879-881.

Jevning R, Wallace RK, Biedebach M. "The physiology of meditation: a review, a wakeful hypometabolic integrated response." *Neuroscience and Biobehavioral Reviews* 1992; 16: 415–424.

Levine, P. "The coherence spectral array (COSPAR) and its application to the study of spatial ordering in the EEG." *Proceedings of the San Diego Biomedical Symposium* 1976; 15: 237–247.

Levine P, Herbert R, Haynes, CT, et al. "EEG coherence during the Transcendental Meditation technique" in *Scientific Research on the Transcendental Meditation Program: Collected Papers,* Vol 1. DW Orme-Johnson DW and JT Farrow (eds). Seelisberg, Switzerland: Maharishi European Research University MIU Press, 1977.

MacLean C, Walton K, Wenneberg S, Levitsky D, Mandarino J, Waziri R, Hillis SL, Schneider RH. "Effects of the Transcendental Meditation program on adaptive mechanisms: changes in hormone levels and responses to stress after 4 months of practice." *Psychoendrocrinology* 1996; 22: 277–295.

Orme-Johnson DW, Farrow JT. *Scientific Research on the Transcendental Meditation Program: Collected Papers,* Vol 1. Seelisberg, Switzerland: Maharishi European Research University MIU Press, 1977.

Orme-Johnson D, Walton K. "All approaches to preventing or reversing effects of stress are not the same." *American Journal of Health Promotion* 1998; 12: 297–299.

Roth, Robert. *Maharishi Mahesh Yogi's TM (Transcendental Meditation)*, Revised and Updated Edition. New York: Donald I. Fine Inc., 1994.

Travis F, Arenander A. "Cross-sectional and longitudinal study of effects of Transcendental Meditation practice on interhemispheric frontal asymmetry and frontal coherence." *International Journal of Neuroscience* (in press).

Chapter 7

Nader T. *Human Physiology: Expression of Veda and the Vedic Literature.* Vlodrop, The Netherlands: MVU Press, 2000.

Schneider RH, Cavanaugh K, Kasture KL, et al. "Health promotion with a traditional system of natural health care: Maharishi Ayur-Veda." *Journal of Social Behavior and Personality* 1990; 5: 1–27.

Sharma, PV, ed. *Caraka Samhita.* Varanasi, India: Chaukahambha Orientalia, 1981.

Chapter 8

Burr M, Buutland B. "Heart disease in British vegetarians." *American Journal of Clinical Nutrition* 1988; 88: 830–832.

Chang-Claude J, Frentzel-Beyme R, Eilber U. "Mortality pattern of German vegetarians after 11 years of follow-up." *Epidemiology* 1992; 3: 395–401.

Fagan, J. *Genetic Engineering—The Hazards. Vedic Engineering: The Solutions.* Fairfield, IA: MUM Press, 1995.

Key TJ, Appleby PN, Davey GK, et al. "Mortality in British vegetarians: review and preliminary results from EPIC-Oxford." *American Journal of Clinical Nutrition* 2003 Sep; 78(3 Suppl): 533S–538S.

Knoops KT, de Groot LC, Kromhout D, et al. "Mediterranean diet, lifestyle factors, and 10-year mortality in elderly European men and women: the HALE project." *Journal of the American Medical Association* 2004; 292: 1490–1492.

Nader T. *Human Physiology—Expression of Veda and the Vedic Literature.* Vlodrop, The Netherlands: MVU Press, 2000.

Ornish D, Brown SE, et al. "Can lifestyle changes reverse coronary heart disease? The Lifestyle Heart Trial." *Lancet* 1990; 336: 624–626.

Schneider RH, Alexander CN, Salerno JW, et al. "Disease prevention and health promotion in the aging with a traditional system of natural medicine: Maharishi Vedic Medicine." *Journal of Aging and Health* 2002; 14: 57–78.

Snowden D. "Animal product consumption and mortality because of all causes combined, coronary heart disease, stroke, diabetes, and cancer in Seventh-Day Adventists." *American Journal of Clinical Nutrition* 1988; 48: 739–748.

Chapter 9

Cullen WJ, Dulchavsky SA, Devasagayam TP, et al. "Effect of Maharishi Amrit Kalash-4 (MAK-4) on H2O2-induced oxidative stress in isolated rat hearts." *Journal of Ethnopharmacology* 1997; 56: 215–222.

Dogra J, Bhargava A. "Lipid peroxide in ischemic heart disease (IHD): inhibition by Maharishi Amrit Kalash (MAK-4 and MAK-5) herbal mixtures." *Federation of the American Societies for Experimental Biology Journal* 2000; 14 (4): A121 (Abstract).

Lee JY, Hanna AN, Lott JA, et al. "The antioxidant and antiatherogenic effects of MAK-4 in WHHL rabbits." *Journal of Alternative and Complementary Medicine* 1996; 2: 463–478.

Lonsdorf N. *The Ageless Woman: Natural Health and Beauty After Forty with Maharishi Ayurveda.* Ann Arbor, MI: MCD Century Publications, 2004.

Niwa Y. "Effect of Maharishi 4 and Maharishi 5 on inflammatory mediators with special reference to their free radical scavenging effect." *Indian Journal of Clinical Practice* 1991; 1: 23–27.

Schneider RH, Alexander CN, Salerno JW, Robinson DK Jr, Fields JZ, et al. "Disease prevention and health promotion in the aging with a traditional system of natural medicine: Maharishi Vedic Medicine." *Journal of Aging and Health* 2002; 14: 57–78.

Sharma HM, Hanna AN, Kauffman EM, et al. "Inhibition of human low-density lipoprotein oxidation in vitro by Maharishi Ayur-Veda herbal mixtures." *Pharmacology Biochemistry and Behavior* 1992; 43: 1175–1182.

Sundaram V, Hanna AN, Lubow GP, et al. "Inhibition of low-density lipoprotein oxidation by oral herbal mixtures Maharishi Amrit Kalash-4 and Maharishi Amrit Kalash-5 in hyperlipidemic patients." *American Journal of the Medical Sciences* 1997: 314: 303–310.

Vohra BP, Sharma SP, Kansal VK. "Effect of Maharishi Amrit Kalash on age dependent variations in mitochondrial antioxidant enzymes, lipid peroxidation and mitochondrial population in different regions of the central nervous system of guinea-pigs." *Drug Metabolism and Drug Interactions* 2001; 18: 57–68

Vohra BP, Sharma SP, Kansal VK, et al. "Effect of Maharishi Amrit Kalash an ayurvedic herbal mixture on lipid peroxidation and neuronal lipofuscin accumulation in ageing guinea pig brain." *Indian Journal of Experimental Biology* 2001; 39: 355–359.

Chapter 10

Hospodar MK. *Heaven's Banquet: Vegetarian Cooking for Lifelong Health the Ayurveda Way*, Plume; Reissue Edition (October 1, 2001).

Chapter 11

Kato M, Phillips B, Sigurdsson G, et al. "Effects of sleep deprivation on neural circulatory control." *Hypertension* 2000; 35: 1173–1175.

Sharma, PV, ed. *Caraka Samhita.* Varanasi, India: Chaukahambha Orientalia, 1981.

Spiegel K, Leproult R, Van Cauter E. "Impact of sleep debt on metabolic and endocrine function." *Lancet* 1999; 354: 1435–1439.

Chapter 12

Herron RE, Fagan JB. "Lipophil-mediated reduction of toxicants in humans: an evaluation of an ayurvedic detoxification procedure." *Alternative Therapies in Health and Medicine* 2002; 8: 40–51.

Schneider RH, Cavanaugh K, Kasture KL, et al. "Health promotion with a traditional system of natural health care: Maharishi Ayur-Veda." *Journal of Social Behavior and Personality* 1990; 5: 1–27.

Sharma HM, Nidich S, Sands D, et al. "Improvements in cardiovascular risk factors through Panchakarma purification procedures." *Journal of Research and Education in Indian Medicine* 1993; 12: 2–13.

Chapter 13

Anderson LM, Fullilove MT, Scrimshaw SC, et al. "Interventions in the social environment to improve community health: a systematic review, systematic review of evidence, recommendations from the Task Force on Community Preventive Services, and Expert Commentary." *American Journal of Preventive Medicine* 2003; 24(3S): 1–80.

Ashton J (ed.): *Healthy Cities.* Milton Keynes, Philadelphia, PA: Open Universities Press, 1992.

Blair HT, Sharp PE. "Anticipatory head direction signals in anterior thalamus." *Journal of Neuroscience* 1995; 15: 6260–6270.

Burge PS. "Sick building syndrome." *Occupational and Environmental Medicine* 2004; 61: 185–190.

Cooke HM, Lynch A. "Biorhythms and chronotherapy in cardiovascular disease." *American Journal of Hospital Pharmacy* 1994; 51: 2569–2580.

Davies JL, Alexander CN. "Alleviating political violence through reducing collective tension: impact assessment analyses of the Lebanon War." *Journal of Social Behavior and Personality* 2005; 17: 285–338.

Diez-Roux AV, Merken SS, Arnet D, et al. "Neighborhood of residence and incidence of coronary heart disease." *New England Journal of Medicine* 2001; 345: 99–106.

Dillbeck MC. "Test of a field theory of consciousness and social change: time-series analysis of participation in the TM-Sidhi program and reduction of violent death." *U.S. Social Indicators Research* 1990; 22: 399–418.

Dillbeck MC, Landrith G, Orme-Johnson DW. "The Transcendental Meditation program and crime rate change in a sample of 48 cities." *Journal of Crime and Justice* 1981; 4: 254–255.

Dunea G. Chronobiology. *British Medical Journal* 1994; 309: 613.

Eyre H, Kahn R, Robertson RM, et al. "Preventing cancer, cardiovascular disease, and diabetes: a common agenda for the American Cancer Society, the American Diabetes Association, and the American heart Association." *Stroke* 2004; 35(8): 1999–2010.

Guo YF, Stein PK. "Circadian rhythm in the cardiovascular system: chronocardiology." *American Heart Journal* 2003; 145: 779–786.

Hagelin JS, Rainforth MV, Orme-Johnson, DW, et al. "Effects of group practice of the Transcendental Meditation program on preventing violent crime in Washington, D.C.: results of the National Demonstration Project, June–July 1993. *Journal of Social Indicators Research* 1999; 47: 153–201.

Healthy Buildings, Healthy People: A Vision for the 21st Century. U.S. Environmental Protection Agency, 402-K01-003, October 2001. http://nepis.epa.gov/Exe/ZyNET.exe/00000323.txt (January 2006). Indoor Air Facts No. 4 (revised): *Sick Building Syndrome (SBS).* US Environmental Protection Agency, Office of Research and Development, April 1991.

Lamberg L. "Medical news and perspectives: dawn's early light to twilight's last gleaming." *Journal of the American Medical Association* 1998; 280: 1556–1558.

Lipman J, Arenander A, Schneider RH. Review of scientific research on Maharishi Vedic Architecture (submitted for publication).

Meisel SR, Kutz I, Dayan KI, et al. "Effect of Iraqi missile war on incidence of acute myocardial infarction and sudden death in Israeli citizens." *Lancet* 1991; 338: 660–661.

Nader T. *Human Physiology: Expression of Veda and the Vedic Literature.* Vlodrop, The Netherlands: MVU Press, 2000.

Orme-Johnson DW. "Medical care utilization and the Transcendental Meditation program." *Psychosomatic Medicine* 1987; 49: 493–507.

Orme-Johnson DW. "Quantifying the field effects of consciousness: from increased EEG coherence to reduced international terrorism." In: Chez RA, editor. *Proceedings: Bridging Worlds and Filling Gaps in the Science of Healing.* Corona del Mar, CA: Samueli Institute for Informational Biology, 2002; 326–346.

Orme-Johnson DW, Alexander CN, Davies JL, et al. "International Peace Project in the Middle East: The effects of the Maharishi technology of the unified field." *Journal of Conflict Resolution* 1988; 32: 776–812.

Pope CA, Burnett RT, Thurston GD, et al. "Cardiovascular mortality and long-term exposure to particulate air pollution: epidemiological evidence of general pathophysiological pathways of disease." *Circulation* 2004; 109: 71–77.

Rajeswari KR, Satyanarayana M, Sanker Narayan PV, et al. "Effect of extremely low frequency magnetic field on serum cholinesterase in humans and animals." *Indian Journal of Experimental Biology* 1985; 23: 194-197.

Redlich C, Sparer J, Cullen MR. "Occupational medicine: Sick building syndrome." *Lancet* 1997; 349: 1013–1016.

Scarpelli P, Gallo M, Chiari G. "Chronobiology of blood pressure." *Journal of Nephrology* 2000; 13: 197–204.

Subrahmanyam S, Sanker Narayan PV, Srinivasan TM. "Effects of low frequency magnetic micropulsations in albino rats." *Biomedicine* 1984; 7: 15–22.

Syme LS, Balfour JL. "Social determinants of Disease" in *Public Health and Preventive Medicine,* edited by RB Wallace and BH Doebbeling. Stamford, CT: Appleton and Lange, 1998.

Tate N. *The Sick Building Syndrome: How Indoor Pollution Is Poisoning Your Life and What You Can Do.* Far Hills, NJ: New Horizon Press, 1994.

Taube JS. "Head direction cells recorded in the anterior thalamic nuclei." *Journal of Neuroscience* 1995; 15: 70–86.

Taube JS, Goodridge JP, Solob EJ, et al. "Processing the head direction cell signal: a review and commentary. *Brain Research Bulletin* 1996; 40: 477–486.

Travis F, Butler B, Rainforth M, et al. "Can a building's orientation affect the quality of life of the people within? Testing principles of Maharishi Sthapatya Veda." *Journal of Social Behavior and Personality* 2005; 17: 533–564.

Weht TA, Rosenthal NE. "Seasonality and affective illness." *American Journal of Psychiatry* 1989; 146: 829–839.

Willett WC. "Balancing life-style and genomics research for disease prevention." *Science* 2002 Apr 26; 296(5568): 695–8.

Chapter 14

Freeman WJ. "Neural networks and chaos." *Journal of Theoretical Biology* 1994; 171: 13–18.

Jason L, Burns MS, et al. "The effects of different types of music on perceived and physiological measures of stress." *Journal of Music Therapy* 2002; 39: 101–116.

Nader T. *Human Physiology: Expression of Veda and the Vedic Literature.* Vlodrop, The Netherlands: MVU Press, 2000.

Nader TA, Smith DE, Dillbeck MC, Schanbacher V, Dillbeck SL, Gallois P, Beall-Rougerie S, Schneider RH, et al. "A double-blind randomized controlled trial of Maharishi Vedic Vibration Technology in subjects with arthritis." *Frontiers in Bioscience* 2001; 6:h7–h17.

Nidich SN, Schneider RH, Nidich RJ, et al. "Maharishi Vedic Vibration Technology on chronic disorders and associated quality of life." *Frontiers in Bioscience* 2001; 6: h1–h6.

Olson TM, Sorflaten JW. "Empirical Investigation of the effects of Maharishi Gandharva Veda Music during live concerts." *Journal of Social Behavior and Personality,* 2005. 17: 571–588.

Sharma HM, Kauffman EM, Stephens RE. "Effect of different sounds on growth of human cancer cell lines in vitro." *Alternative Therapies in Clinical Practice* 1996; 3: 25–32.

Talbott E, Hemkamp J, Matthews K, et al. "Occupational noise exposure, noise induced hearing loss, and the epidemiology of high blood pressure." *American Journal of Epidemiology* 1985; 121: 501–514.

Chapter 15

Alexander CN, Langer E, Newman RI, et al. "Enhancing health and longevity: the Transcendental Meditation program, mindfulness, and the elderly." *Journal of Personality and Social Psychology* 1989; 57: 950–964.

Fields JZ, Walton KG, Schneider RH, et al. "Effect of a multi-modality natural medicine program on carotid atherosclerosis in older subjects: A pilot trial of Maharishi Vedic Medicine." *American Journal of Cardiology* 2002; 89: 952–958.

Nader T, Averbach R, Charles B, Fields JZ, Schneider RH. "Improvements in chronic diseases with a comprehensive natural medicine approach: a review and case series." *Behavioral Medicine* 2000; 26: 34–46.

Orme-Johnson DW, Herron RE. "An innovative approach to reducing medical care utilization and expenditures." *American Journal of Managed Care* 1997; 3: 135–144.

Rothenberg S, Belok S, Fields JZ. "The Maharishi Vedic Medicine Chronic Disorders Program, introduction and case histories." *Alternative & Complementary Therapies* 2003; 9: 183–190.

Schneider RH, Alexander C, Salerno J, et al. "Disease prevention and health promotion in the aging with a traditional system of natural medicine: Maharishi Vedic Medicine." *Journal of Aging and Health* 2002; 14: 57–78.

Wallace RK, Dillbeck M, Jacobe E, et al. "The effects of the Transcendental Meditation and TM-Sidhi program on the aging process." *International Journal of Neuroscience* 1982; 16: 53–58.

Index

About the Authors

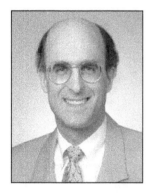

Robert H. Schneider, M.D., F.A.C.C., is a physician, scientist, educator, and one of the world's leading authorities on natural medicine and its scientific use in the prevention and treatment of heart disease. Over the past twenty years, he has directed nearly $20 million in research grants from the National Institutes of Health for his pioneering research on natural approaches to heart disease. The results of this groundbreaking research have been published in more than 100 articles in authoritative medical journals and proceedings, and featured in more than 1,000 television, radio, magazine, and newspaper reports, including ABC's *20/20, CNN Headline News, Fox News,* the *New York Times, Washington Post, Newsweek, Wall Street Journal,* and *Time* magazine.

Dr. Schneider is board-certified in preventive medicine, is a certified specialist in clinical hypertension and a Fellow of the American College of Cardiology. He did his postgraduate training in internal medicine and hypertension at the University of Michigan Medical School. He has been a consultant to numerous government agencies, including to the National Institutes of Health (NIH), the Centers for Disease Control and Prevention, the Presidential Commission on Complementary and Alternative Medicine, and the U.S. Congress' Prevention Coalition. Dr. Schneider is a frequent lecturer on natural health care at medical centers and professional societies on four continents.

Currently, Dr. Schneider is the director of the NIH-funded Institute for Natural Medicine and Prevention and professor of physiology and health at Maharishi University of Management.

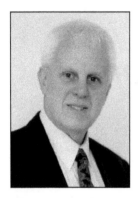

Jeremy Z. Fields, Ph.D., (pharmacology) has more than thirty years of experience in NIH- and VA-funded biomedical research, including work in the field of evidence-based, prevention-oriented natural medicine. He has published extensively in the peer-reviewed scientific literature. In addition, Dr. Fields is an experienced professional science writer and editor. He has held faculty positions at Chicago Medical School and Loyola Medical School–Chicago. He lives in Freeport, Maine.